*Love, Money, and HIV*

# Love, Money, and HIV

## BECOMING A MODERN AFRICAN WOMAN IN THE AGE OF AIDS

Sanyu A. Mojola

UNIVERSITY OF CALIFORNIA PRESS

University of California Press, one of the most distinguished university presses in the United States, enriches lives around the world by advancing scholarship in the humanities, social sciences, and natural sciences. Its activities are supported by the UC Press Foundation and by philanthropic contributions from individuals and institutions. For more information, visit www.ucpress.edu.

University of California Press
Oakland, California

Library of Congress Cataloging-in-Publication Data

Mojola, Sanyu A., 1979– author.
    Love, money, and HIV : becoming a modern African woman in the age of AIDS / Sanyu A. Mojola.
        page   cm.
    Includes bibliographical references and index.
    ISBN 978–0–520–28093–9 (cloth : alk. paper)
    ISBN 978–0–520–28094–6 (pbk. : alk. paper)
    ISBN 978–0–520–95850–0 (ebook)
    1. Young women—Health risk assessment—Kenya—Nyanza Province.   2. Young women—Sexual behavior—Kenya—Nyanza Province.   3. Young women—Kenya—Nyanza Province—Economic conditions.   4. Young women—Africa, Sub-Saharan—Economic conditions.   5. HIV infections—Sex factors—Kenya—Nyanza Province.   6. HIV infections—Sex factors—Africa, Sub-Saharan.   7. AIDS (Disease)—Risk factors—Kenya—Nyanza Province.   8. AIDS (Disease)—Risk factors—Africa, Sub-Saharan.   9. AIDS (Disease) in women—Africa, Sub-Saharan—Prevention.   10. Women consumers—Africa, Sub-Saharan—Attitudes. I. Title.
    RA643.86.K42N936   2014
    362.1084220967—dc23                                        2013041589

23   22   21   20   19   18   17   16   15   14
10   9   8   7   6   5   4   3   2   1

To Papa, Mummy, Luka, and Wanga, for loving, encouraging, and believing in me.

To Kukhu Yuniya Aluoch and Jajja Gertrude Kiyingi, my grandmothers, two amazing and inspiring women. I am grateful to have reached this far in my education during their lifetimes, and that they have lived long enough to hold this book in their hands.

# Contents

# Illustrations

TABLES

# Preface

Becoming ill is not just a random event. I still remember sitting in David Byrne's Sociology of Health class while pursuing my undergraduate degree at Durham University in the north of England and being struck by that revelation. As the class progressed, there were more. Sociologists, demographers, and epidemiologists, I learned, could *predict* which groups of people in a given society would get sick and which would die early. Further, there was often a highly organized social-structural pattern to disease and mortality, above and beyond seemingly random and idiosyncratic individual choices—about who to love, or where to work, or which tap to collect water from—that led to illness and death. Coming from a continent plagued by one disease after another, I found these ideas revolutionary. In the decade and a half that followed, these ideas began to shape how I saw and understood the HIV/AIDS epidemic in Africa, and how I thought about how to end it.

When I graduated from Durham and returned home to Dodoma, Tanzania, where my family and I lived at the time, I interned for a few months at the AIDS control agency of the Anglican Church of Tanzania, under the program officer Neema Peter. The experience was both revealing and frustrating. It was revealing to see that most of our clients were women, who were processing the outcomes of HIV tests without any hope of treatment, and to see the gaps that existed between knowledge and behavior. It was frustrating to realize that while the one-by-one, community-by-community approach was vitally important, the problem of HIV/AIDS in Africa, and among women in particular, required an approach that would help *millions*.

It was partly impatience—for a structural approach, for something that would help the millions—that led me to apply, with my father's encouragement, to graduate school in America (where funding was available for graduate students), to take up the fellowship that the University of Chicago offered, and to stay through the long and grueling years that followed in dogged pursuit of my doctorate in sociology. That journey was circuitous; it involved my dipping into courses across several disciplines, including sociology, demography, public policy, social epidemiology, economics, anthropology, history, and political science as I tried to gather enough information and analytical and practical tools to begin to investigate the problem of HIV/AIDS in Africa and figure out what to do about it. It has taken more years and greater patience than I ever imagined to finally have something to say.

It is my hope that this book reinvigorates ambitious thinking regarding the HIV/AIDS pandemic in Africa, not just thinking that focuses on the important task of improving and prolonging lives, but creative thinking about how to bring the epidemic to an end. In doing so, I hope it does justice to my respondents, whose voices and insights fill these pages, as well as my fellow Africans more broadly, who deserve a chance to live an HIV-free life and to navigate their sexual and romantic lives without the specter of illness and death hanging over them.

*Sanyu Amimo Mojola*
*Boulder, Colorado*
*September 2013*

# 1  A Stubborn Disparity

The bustling city of Kisumu, the capital of Nyanza province, Kenya, lies nestled by Lake Victoria, the largest freshwater lake in Africa, and only a few miles from the equator. A stroll through its main streets yields a display of an apparent clash of worlds and cultures. There is the Africa we know: the busy human drama of *mitumba* (secondhand clothing) women, market traders and hawkers, street children, fishermen and the pungent smell of fresh and smoking fish, house flies and mosquitos, numerous bicycles and *matatus* (public transportation vehicles) hooting through the town, and travelers stopping by on the way to or from Uganda or Tanzania. And there is the Africa we are coming to know: tarmaced streets, a prominent Citibank building (taken up by another company), Internet cafes, international nongovernmental organizations (NGOs), and English billboards prominently advertising pay-as-you-go Safaricom mobile phones and Trust condoms. The exuberance, color, and activity of Kisumu, however, mask the slow and terrible unfolding of a demographic catastrophe. A survey conducted in the late 1990s revealed that, among its young women, almost 30% of 15–19 year olds and almost 40% of 20–24 year olds were HIV positive, carrying a virus that would kill them in six to ten years. These were three to six times the HIV rates of same-aged men.[1]

Unfortunately, the gender disparities in this survey were not unique to Kisumu, Kenya, but were reflected in study after study across sub-Saharan Africa, the world's most affected region. Despite having only 12% of the world's population, it has 69% (23.5 million) of people living with HIV/AIDS, 70% (1.2 million) of AIDS-related deaths, and 71% (1.8 million) of new infections.[2]

Women now make up approximately 60% of Africans living with HIV/AIDS,[3] and young women are at particular risk. In 2001, in *AIDS*, the official journal of the International AIDS Society, an influential editorial comment was published with the title, "To Stem HIV in Africa, Prevent Transmission to Young Women." The authors noted that "the high HIV prevalence among women aged 15–19 years could be critical in provoking and maintaining an explosive HIV epidemic."[4] The editorial concluded by urging policy makers to focus their efforts on this group of young people. The issue becomes much more salient in light of the current burgeoning youth population in sub-Saharan Africa: 41% of Africans are under age 15.[5] Girls in this demographic group are on the brink of their greatest period of risk of contracting HIV. This situation offers both an extraordinary opportunity to halt the epidemic and potential disaster if the HIV epidemic is not stemmed.[6]

Despite the early call for action, gender differences in HIV rates among youth in sub-Saharan Africa continue to be widespread and have been confirmed over the subsequent decade in several larger and more representative surveys than those that prompted the comment. Further, these disparities tend to persist until youth reach their mid-30s; after that point, we start to see substantial variation by country in which gender has higher HIV rates.[7]

Figure 1, for example, shows findings from a sample of national surveys of HIV-prevalence rates among young men and women in selected high-prevalence countries in sub-Saharan Africa. It illustrates not only the high burden of HIV in countries such as South Africa, which holds the world's largest HIV-positive population (over five million people), but also the *variability* across countries in the size of the disparity between young men and women. In South Africa, 31% of 21-year-old women are HIV positive, a rate that is five times higher than same-aged men, who have a prevalence rate of 5.6%. However, in Zimbabwe, 15–19-year-old females'

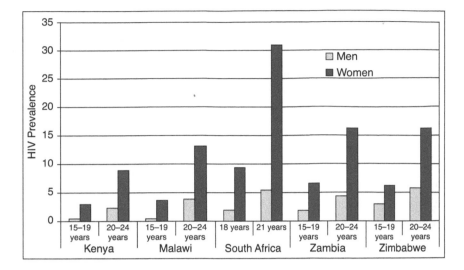

*Figure 1.* HIV prevalence among young men and women in sub-Saharan Africa.
Sources: KDHS 2004; MDHS 2005; Pettifor et al. 2005; ZDHS 2003; ZDHS 2007.

6.2% HIV prevalence is only twice as high as same-aged men, who have a prevalence rate of 3.1%. On average, young African women are three times more likely than young men to have HIV;[8] however, as the figure illustrates, this average masks widely varying levels of disproportionate risk. Indeed, this variability in youth-gender disparities across the region suggests that this is not merely a story of biological sex differences. Something more is at work.

## A LIFE-COURSE APPROACH TO HIV RISK

The *youth*-gender disparity from ages 15 to 24 matters because young women have so much more to lose than men in years of life that are disease free and in life expectancy. As figure 1 illustrates, substantial numbers of people are contracting HIV on the cusp of adulthood. In the absence of antiretroviral medication, many are dying early in their marriages, leaving behind young children. For men, not only are they acquiring HIV at lower rates than women in their adolescence and early adulthood, but their peak

HIV prevalence is also much later, in their late 30s or early 40s. This means that they lose far fewer years relative to their life expectancy compared to women.[9] An important place to start, then, in investigating the gender disparity in HIV rates is to investigate the period in the life course when these disparities emerge and self-perpetuate—the transition to adulthood.

A "transition-to-adulthood" framework provides a lens through which to examine social processes and experiences salient to youth in the period between puberty and adulthood. It is a useful way of exploring the lives and developmental changes and challenges experienced by African youth by allowing the examination of key transitions such as relationship formation processes (including sexual initiation and the culmination of relationships in marriage or a stable partnership), the pursuit of education, finding employment, attaining financial independence, becoming a parent, and transitioning residences (principally moving out of the parental home).[10] Importantly, these life-course transitions *co-occur:* relationship decisions can be shaped by educational decisions; financial independence can determine residential transition.[11] This co-occurrence of many life-changing and life-impacting decisions creates for young people a thick web of life events that is reflected in the fact that many experience their transition to adulthood as complicated and confusing. Because of the life-long significance of many decisions made during this period, transitions to adulthood are sometimes characterized as *risky.* This recognizes the fact that mistimed (early or delayed), missed, or unsuccessful transitions to "normal" adulthood, or events and actions that interrupt an otherwise smooth transition, can have potentially long-term implications for educational attainment, lifetime income, job prospects, and health. Substance abuse, juvenile delinquency, teenage pregnancy, and HIV, for example, can complicate or even derail a young person's successful transition to adulthood by limiting their ability to enact other transitions such as finding employment, achieving financial independence, and forming stable long-term relationships.

Additionally, it is important to acknowledge that transitions have a *processual* nature. In other words, the establishing of a stable long-term relationship (and even parenthood), the completion of education, and stable employment are all transitions that can be begun, ended, elongated, interrupted, restarted, and returned to.[12] My interest in a life-course approach, and the transition-to-adulthood perspective in particular, is to examine not so much the point at which adulthood is reached (though this is touched on), but rather the *process* of its attainment. This facilitates an analytical strategy that uses a focus on various transitions to adulthood to bring into relief the ways in which gender disparities in HIV rates emerge and are produced among young people.

## THE BOOK

The consistently higher HIV rates of young women across a subcontinent with diverse countries, cultures, and ethnic groups belie a phenomenon that is only captured by biological sex differences or a patchwork of localized stories. Rather, it suggests that overarching social-structural processes are *also* occurring across the continent, mapping onto biology, individual decision-making, and culture in local spaces. The combination of these processes places young African women transitioning to adulthood at great risk, while producing temporary safety for young men. At the heart of this book is a study of how one of these processes—consumption, the desire for and purchasing of modern goods—has come to play a crucial role in producing gendered life and death outcomes among young people.

The startling statistics cited at the beginning of this chapter struck a deep personal chord as a Kenyan native with a paternal grandmother from Nyanza province, who I regularly visited during school holidays. These were not distant statistics. They numerically represented a demographic category I inhabited. The age group, gender, and ethnic heritage of those at the highest risk at the time of the survey perfectly characterized me as well as several female cousins living in or near Kisumu, Nyanza's capital. Further investigation of the statistics revealed that young African women were at greater risk compared not just to men in Nyanza province, but to men in almost every African country for which I could find data. Why were young African women at much greater risk for HIV compared to same-aged young men? Biology was clearly part of the explanation, but the *variation* in the disparity from setting to setting suggested that something more was going on, something that I felt survey analysis alone could not quite capture. I designed a mixed-methods study to explore this disparity. Drawing on a life-course framework, the study explored young people's transitions to adulthood in the context of an ongoing HIV epidemic, drawing on the perspectives of 185 young people, middle-aged adults, and older adults, as well as 20 key informants. Rather than abandoning quantitative data, I chose to move back and forth between population-based survey data from Kenya, ethnographic and interview-based fieldwork in Nyanza province, Kenya (the setting that launched my interest in this topic), and published quantitative and qualitative analyses from several parts of sub-Saharan Africa in order to come to a more complete understanding not only of the plight of young women in Nyanza, but also of those living in many other parts of the continent.

This book examines how young African women navigate their relationships, schooling, employment, and financial access in the context of a devastating HIV epidemic and economic inequality, where extreme wealth is increasing alongside extreme poverty. Billboards in rural and urban sub-Saharan Africa advertising modern lifestyles and consumer products are an indelible part of the social landscape. This means that modernity and the consumptive goods and practices that signify it are present and highly visible in many rapidly globalizing parts of the continent, but just out of reach for many.[13] These developments are deeply gendered and have implications for young women's HIV rates. The book examines the compounding of young women's desire for consumer products that require continual replenishment with the gendered and generational nature of access to income as well as resources. Many young African women are situated within stages in their life course and social structures where access to money, resources, and paid work is tightly constrained. Continual consumption requires partners with continual access to income. This ultimately makes intimate relationships with older, employed men, who have higher HIV-prevalence rates, more attractive than those with unemployed young men, who have relatively low HIV rates.

Let us briefly listen in on a conversation typical of the many I had with groups of high school girls in Nyanza. We had been talking about who they most saw affected by HIV/AIDS, and they said it was young women. I asked them why, and the following unfolded:

SANYU: Why do you think it's mostly girls? Why not boys?

ANYANGO: Because girls are being attracted to so many things.

MARY: They are easily swayed by money.

SACHA: This is because of the financial status of the family, whereby if the family is poor, you know as girls we need several things, but if the family can't provide all this, the girl will be forced to search for them somewhere else, and if you find somebody who cannot provide all these necessities, the girl may switch to the next man she thinks might provide it. So that's the reason as to why the girls move from one man to another, and get infected to this disease easier.

SANYU: So what things do girls need? It's been a while since I was in high school.

JANE: Cosmetics, maybe your friends look smarter than you . . .

ROSA: Good dresses.

ANYANGO: And she doesn't have . . .

SACHA: Which will force you to search for a man who can provide all this. *[Laughter.]*

SANYU: So that means it can't be a fellow guy in high school? 'Cause he doesn't have the money? Or does it not matter? *[Silence.]*

ROSA: It must just be somebody from, someone who is financially stable, who can provide for all this.

SANYU: And what age would that be . . . someone not in school?

JANE: No, those in the working class.

In thinking through this and many other such conversations, a number of things became apparent. First, their knowledge about the epidemic was not lacking. They were aware that their demographic—young women—had the most risk for HIV, and further, they were aware that they could get HIV from sexual relationships, with the most risk coming from having multiple partners. Second, they were clear that the reason why girls were most at risk was because of their desire for *nonsurvival* consumption, and that it was men who worked—"working-class" men—who were most able to provide them with the money to consume. The fact that things like cosmetics and good dresses were framed as *necessities* or needs led to a compulsion, indeed something that would "force" them to look for a man to help.

Many elements of this conversation are familiar to Africanist and AIDS scholars, who have similarly observed and written about transactional sex relationships—intimate relationships where money and gifts are exchanged but in which issues of love and trust are also considered at stake. However, few have moved beyond discussing the nature of these relationships to unpacking why young African women want to consume in the first place. In other words, while much is known about the existence and widespread nature of these relationships, little is known about *why* and importantly *how* young women across the continent have historically come to desire consumption to this degree, despite widespread knowledge about HIV/AIDS and widespread experience of the emotional and social devastation that has accompanied it. In using a mixed-methods approach to examining how girls transform into "consuming women" as they transition into adulthood, this book will not only unpack these puzzles, but also, in the process, shed light on three startling quantitative paradoxes in the AIDS literature that are part of the problem of young women's disproportionate HIV risk: why women living in the wealthiest households in Africa have the highest rates of HIV (chapters 2, 4, and 5), why the least-educated African women have the lowest rates of HIV (chapter 5), and why African women who work for pay have higher rates of HIV compared to those who do not (chapter 6). Bringing to the fore the voices, thoughts, and experiences of young African women and men in the chapters that follow, along with representative survey data, this book will show how the complicated entanglement of love, money, and young women's transformation into "consuming women" lies at the heart of their disproportionate HIV rates.

The book examines how desires for money, gifts, modernity, and consumption become both gendered—with girls constructed as desiring more than boys—and inextricably linked with girls' intimate relationships with the riskiest male partners. Specifically, I illustrate how consuming young women have been *cultivated* and *produced* in three contexts—communities, schools, and labor markets. I explore the historical and contemporary construction of "gendered needs"—young women's continual and disproportionately greater "needs" for modern products that must be bought, such as sanitary pads, cosmetics, and clothing compared to young men. I then situate these desires in three social-structural contexts: in communities, where the means of achieving beauty and attracting partners have over time become commodified (chapters 3 and 4); in schools, which are settings charged with the production of modern subjects, a modernity that young women's consuming practices signify (chapter 5); and in gendered labor markets, where the gap between young women's "needs" and their access to money, resources, and paid work becomes particularly acute, and where transactional relationships take on new significance (chapter 6). In the case of gendered labor markets, I further show how changing ecological environments mapped onto gendered economies can shape the sexual economies in which transactional relationships unfold with devastating effects on young women's HIV risk.

In the rest of this chapter, I first review the literature on gender differences in youth HIV rates, and then discuss the setting, data, and methods used in the study before concluding with a brief overview of the chapters in this book.

## GENDER DIFFERENCES IN YOUTH HIV RATES

An extensive literature has emerged to examine factors that might explain why young women have higher HIV rates than young men. These factors can be loosely grouped into three sets of explanations: biophysiological, proximate, and social structural. However, many of these explanations not only are limited in their ability to account for the stubborn gender disparity in youth HIV rates across Africa's varied settings, but also suggest particular vulnerability not just for young women, but also for young men. A secondary aim of this section is to introduce readers who may be less familiar with the HIV/AIDS literature to some of the key factors underlying its spread.

### Biophysiological Explanations

A particularly compelling explanation for the disparity in HIV risk between young men and women is young women's higher biophysiological susceptibility to the virus.[14] The HIV virus is contracted through exposure to four transmitting fluids: semen, vaginal fluid, blood, and breast milk, with the highest concentrations of the HIV virus occurring in blood and semen. In sub-Saharan Africa, most young women's HIV risk is the result of exposure to HIV through heterosexual intercourse.[15] Even if a young woman has only one sexual partner, there are several biophysiological reasons why she might be at greater risk of contracting HIV compared to a young man. For example, there is a higher viral load in semen compared to vaginal secretions. Additionally, young women's bodies are particularly vulnerable when they are still developing, and they thus are more likely to experience genital trauma during sex that may create more openings for the virus to enter. The presence of blood when virginity is lost is also likely to place young women at higher risk of contracting HIV compared to young men.

However, findings on sex differences in transmission probabilities of HIV are mixed. While many studies from Europe and the United States suggest greater male-female transmission probabilities (that is, a man is more likely to transmit HIV to a woman), results from developing countries such as Thailand, Kenya, and Uganda suggest the opposite trend. These studies suggest that women have higher transmission probabilities than men and are more likely to transmit HIV to men than vice versa. Part of the explanation for this is that men in developing countries are more likely to have high-risk partners such as commercial sex workers. Because commercial sex workers have many sexual partners, they are a population that is particularly vulnerable to being exposed to HIV, as well as to passing HIV on to others. Sex workers also have a higher likelihood of being exposed to other sexually transmitted infections (STIs).[16] Having an STI increases the likelihood of contracting HIV because STIs create additional openings for HIV to enter and may also increase the amount of HIV in vaginal fluids, thus increasing women's transmission probabilities.[17]

Uncircumcised men also experience higher HIV risk compared to men who are circumcised. Many of the countries and ethnic groups greatly affected by the HIV epidemic have lower male circumcision rates.[18] In the most thorough confirmation of this finding, researchers enrolled several hundred men in Kenya, South Africa, and Uganda, randomly divided them into two groups, and circumcised one group, while leaving the other group intact. Following them over several months, they found significantly lower HIV rates among the men who were circumcised in all three countries. In Kenya, for example, men from Kisumu, the town profiled at the beginning of the chapter, who were circumcised experienced a 53%

reduced risk of acquiring HIV compared to the men who had been left intact. Biological studies also suggest that circumcised men face reduced risk for the acquisition of ulcerative STIs, which appear to greatly exacerbate the risk of acquiring HIV.[19] Transmission probabilities, STI acquisition, and the lack of circumcision are all factors that suggest vulnerability for young African men. In sum, while biophysiological factors clearly play a role, they are not in and of themselves sufficient explanations for young women's consistently higher prevalence levels across sub-Saharan Africa. Further, biology does not explain the *variance* in gender differences in HIV rates. Why, for example, were Zimbabwean women twice as vulnerable as their male counterparts, while South African women were five times as vulnerable, as shown in figure 1?

## Proximate Explanations

Since heterosexual intercourse is a central mode of HIV transmission in Africa, perhaps how different cultures and ethnicities shape the proximate determinants of the sexual acquisition of HIV is the most important factor.[20] These factors directly affect (1) how much infected sexual fluid an individual is likely to be exposed to, and (2) how risky that exposure is. Exposure to infected fluid can be examined through factors such as age at first sex (affecting length of sexual activity) and number of sexual partners (and partners' partners). The risk of exposure can be examined through factors such as frequency of condom use (the most effective means of preventing sexual HIV transmission).

### AGE AT FIRST SEX

A particularly consequential factor that might be affected by culture is the age at which an individual begins sex. In addition to the presence of blood at first sex, an early sexual debut also affects the length of time an individual has been sexually active and potentially exposed to HIV. For example, in Nyanza province, while men's median age at first sex is 17.4 years, women begin sex almost half a year earlier at 16.7 years.[21] This means that women experience a longer duration of potential exposure to HIV compared to men, which may partially underlie their higher HIV rates. However, in other parts of Africa with high HIV prevalence, this factor seems less important. In Manicaland, Zimbabwe, for example, the median age at sexual debut was *the same* for men and women (18.5 years) despite the 20%–25% difference in HIV prevalence rates. In South Africa, men begin sex *earlier* than women, despite young women's having five times the HIV rates of same-aged young men.[22]

## AGE AND NUMBER OF SEXUAL PARTNERS

The more sexual partners an individual has, the greater their chance of encountering an HIV positive partner. This would also be a compelling explanation for young women's higher rates except for the fact that young men typically report *more* sexual partners than young women.[23] Women's primary risk occurs because their fewer reported partners are typically older, and in some cases considerably older than they are. While young women have higher HIV rates than *same-aged* men, in many settings they have *lower* HIV rates than men five to ten years older. Thus a 17-year-old female with only one 25-year-old sexual partner is more likely to be exposed to HIV than another same-aged female with three 17-year-old sexual partners.[24] However, one could also make the opposite argument. Young men's sexual partners are highly risky partners; their female counterparts aged 15 and above have higher HIV rates than them. Thus young men's likelihood of encountering an HIV-infected same-aged partner would actually be *higher* than that of a young woman. So to the extent that a young man is sexually active, his same-aged partners are of far greater risk to him than he is to them.

## CONDOM USE

These relationships would not be as risky if every sexual act was protected by condom use, the most effective method of prevention of sexually transmitted HIV (aside from abstinence). While condom use has increased significantly over the past few years and knowledge of condoms was over 85% in several sub-Saharan African countries, in most of these countries, only about a third to a half of sexually active young men aged 15–29 reported condom use at last sex. Older, and especially married, men's condom use is dramatically lower, as is self-reported use among young women. The abiding problem for many public health officials working on HIV interventions in sub-Saharan Africa is the continued resistance to widespread and consistent condom use before, within, and out of marriage.[25]

*Connective Social-Structural Explanations*

These are some of the major proximate explanations underlying young women's higher HIV risk, and they are useful to varying degrees in understanding the phenomenon in particular cultures, settings, and countries. However, they are incomplete in explaining why young women's greater HIV risk is replicated across so many diverse settings in sub-Saharan Africa despite different combinations of factors, some of which seem to clearly disadvantage young men more than young women. It does not seem to matter what unique configuration of these factors are operating in a given locale—young women still have higher HIV rates compared to young men.

This stubborn gender disparity in youth HIV rates suggests that there are common overarching social-structural processes at work across a number of settings that are connecting multi-level factors together in similar ways. Connective social-structural processes *organize* biophysiological and proximate determinants of HIV risk in similar ways, and thus can account for similar gendered and generational outcomes across multiple geographic spaces and cultures. Two of the most prominent connective social-structural processes discussed in the literature are sexual networks and migration.

SEXUAL NETWORKS

The study of sexual networks involves capturing a bird's-eye view of structural patterns of sexual relationships in particular communities, enabling an examination not only of an individual's sexual relationships, but also of the relationships of their sexual partners' partners, ultimately revealing how individuals are connected to other individuals through sexual relationships. Thus studies have mapped entire romantic and sexual networks within a US high school and on an island in Malawi, for example.[26] Such studies make visible the HIV risk a young woman may have even if she is monogamous. For example, in figure 2, Liz only has a single sexual partner, Tom. However, Tom is also having concurrent sexual partnerships with Jane and Crystal. Crystal is HIV positive and transmitted HIV to her husband, Jim. In this sexual network, then, Liz is at great risk of HIV acquisition because her sexual partner's partner Crystal is HIV positive. If Tom continues his relationship with Crystal without protection, over time, he will get HIV, which he might then pass on to Liz as well as

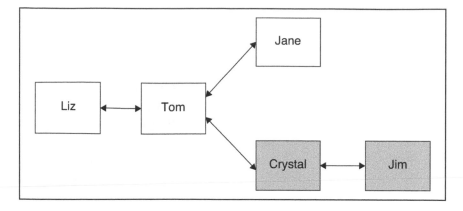

*Figure 2.* Example of a sexual network. Arrows indicate sexual relationships. Dark boxes indicate HIV-positive status.

Jane. In this way, HIV can spread through a sexual network, affecting many people in a short space of time.

In this case, Liz may not be aware that Tom is being unfaithful and may not think she is at risk. However, in many settings across the continent, men's concurrent partnerships are normalized, culturally accepted, and even institutionalized.[27] The most common institutionalized form of concurrency is polygamy where men can legally (as recognized by the state through customary law) have more than one wife. Outside of or in addition to this, informal arrangements ("outside" wives or mistresses) are also common.[28] Thus one HIV-infected man can pass HIV on to his wives and extramarital or nonmarital partners, ultimately contributing to larger numbers of infected women relative to men.[29] These features of sexual networks appear in several settings across the continent.

However, women can also place men at risk through their own concurrent partnerships. A study analyzing population-based representative surveys with HIV sero-discordant couples (where one member is HIV positive and the other HIV negative) found that, in 30%–40% of cases, women were the HIV-positive partners.[30] This suggests that the case of Crystal in figure 2 is not rare. However, when we take a life-course perspective to HIV risk, young women like Liz may be acquiring HIV in a premarital relationship, and then getting married to a man with more than one wife, thus introducing HIV into the sexual network. In these ways, then, women's pre- or extramarital relationships with high-risk partners (such as older men) or multiple partners can also place their marital partners at high risk of acquiring HIV. Additionally, from a cross-sectional perspective, more men than women may be involved in concurrent partnerships overall, thus putting multiple women at risk for HIV at a single point in time. However, from a life-course or longitudinal perspective, young women's concurrency, such as that of Crystal, both during premarital relationships and entering into polygamous first marriages as junior wives, may also be placing multiple men at risk for HIV.[31]

MIGRATION

Migration and mobility are also key connective social-structural processes that have facilitated the rapid spread of HIV across large spaces in Africa. Migration essentially puts sexual networks in motion. Much of the Southern African epidemic, it is argued, is rooted in colonial-era labor migration systems still in place today, which separate workers from their families with only periodic returns home.[32] At either end, opportunities for concurrent relationships exist for *both* men and women. Male workers living in single-sex residential environments seek sexual relief among commercial sex workers or engage in longer-term relationships with women in their work environments. Meanwhile at home, wives and partners might stray for loneliness, or, in some cases, they might seek economic support if their husbands do not send money home. Unprotected partnerships at each end provide ample opportunity for HIV infection to be acquired and then passed on to a partner during reunions.

Along with this, HIV-prevalence rates are particularly high among other kinds of people who are occupationally mobile. Commercial truck drivers who transport goods along major trade routes across Africa, for example, have been found to have particularly high HIV-prevalence rates and, to some extent, serve as vectors for the disease, engaging in relationships with women at different truck stops along Trans-African highways.[33] However, these women might also serve as bridges of disease transmission between high-risk truckers and the local populations in which they reside, an important sexual-network link in epidemics.[34] In addition to the highways, several of the areas hardest and earliest hit by HIV in Kenya (Nyanza province), Uganda (Rakai district), and Tanzania (Mwanza province) lie around Lake Victoria, Africa's largest freshwater lake and the source of the Nile, another major space across which goods are transported and traded. Fishing communities—men and women alike—have been particularly devastated by HIV.[35]

Other potential vectors of the disease are large-scale movements of armies, rebels, and refugees as a result of regional conflict,[36] as well as the voluntary, commercial, and coercive sexual encounters that often follow. HIV transmission in these settings is fueled by the widespread presence of STIs (as noted earlier, an important cofactor of HIV), reflecting poor public sexual-health systems, which often break down in times of war.[37] Young men seeking economic opportunity in mines or major towns, as well as young soldiers and rebels, may engage in high-risk behavior while away from their wives and partners. Many young women may be dependent on remittances or relationships with resident men for access to income, or they may be vulnerable to sexual violence as refugees or victims of conflict. These factors, in combination, imply risk for *both* young men and women.

In this book, I focus on another connective social-structural process, one that emerged as key to more clearly explaining gender differences in HIV outcomes among young people: consumption. Specifically, I show (1) how consumption desires and practices differentially shaped young women's and men's individual sexual decision-making, thus directly affecting their proximate determinants of HIV risk, (2) how consumption operated at a social-structural level within institutions such as schools and labor markets to shape the environments and structure of the sexual networks in which young women in particular were making these decisions, and finally (3) the similarity of these gendered and sexual economy dynamics across several high-prevalence settings throughout sub-Saharan Africa. In the remaining portion of this chapter, I discuss the setting, data, and methodology used in this study, and provide a brief overview of the book's chapters.

STUDY SETTING

Kenya is an East African country, 582,646 square kilometers large, that lies along the Indian Ocean, and is bordered by South Sudan, Somalia, and Ethiopia to its north, Uganda to its west, and Tanzania to its south. A former British colony, it gained independence in 1963, led by its first president, Jomo Kenyatta. Kenya has had three presidents since then; the most recent, Uhuru Kenyatta, the son of the first president, was elected in March 2013. Kenya is considered a low-income country. It ranks 145th out of 186 on the human development index; it has an annual GDP of $33.6 billion and a GNI of $1541 per capita. Almost half the country (46%) lives on or under the poverty line ($1.25 a day). About 24% of the population lives in urban areas, and about 87% of the adult population are literate. In the census from 2010, the country's population was estimated at 39.4 million people. The country has a 2.7% annual rate of population growth with a total fertility rate of 4.6 children per woman.[38]

Kenya is divided into eight provinces. Nyanza, the site of this study, which is located in the west, is the third most populous, with 5.4 million residents, about 14% of the country's population. The Luo are a Nilotic ethnic group primarily living in Nyanza. They are the third largest ethnic group in the country, following the Kikuyu and the Luhya ethnic groups. While several studies have been undertaken in this area over the past decade, and while a lot of money has been spent, many communication campaigns have been mounted, and several nongovernmental organizations (NGOs) have invested in fighting HIV in Nyanza, the epidemic persists.[39] Why this is the case remains a mystery. Nyanza also provides an example of a province with macroeconomic elements common to other parts of Africa that are affected by HIV: it is a labor-migrating province, situated along major trading routes, including the Trans-African highway. However, despite large volumes of trade passing through Nyanza, many of its inhabitants remain poor. District Development Plans for the districts in this study recorded absolute poverty rates (proportions of people living on less than $1 a day) ranging from 53% to 69%, making it one of the poorest provinces in the country. In Kenya as a whole, 8% of women and 4.3% of men were HIV positive. However, as figure 3 illustrates, Nyanza province has the highest rates in the country. One in six women (16%) and one in ten men (11.4%) are HIV positive. The Luo ethnic group also has the highest HIV rates in the province,[40] as well as in the country as a whole. One in five Luo women (22.8%) and one in six Luo men (17.1%) are HIV positive (figure 4).[41]

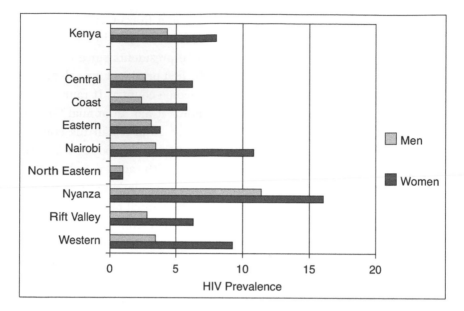

*Figure 3.* HIV prevalence by province. Source: KDHS 2010.

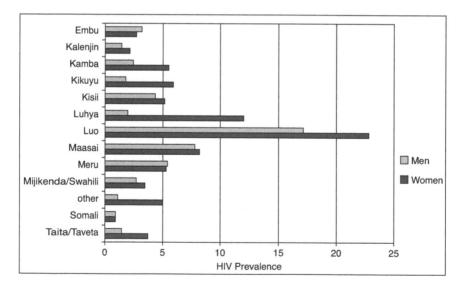

*Figure 4.* HIV prevalence by ethnic group. Source: KDHS 2010.

Studying the epidemic among the Luo in Nyanza province is particularly significant because it is in the region where the HIV epidemic began and that has borne the HIV/AIDS epidemic the longest. After HIV became an epidemic in Central Africa in the late 1970s, the disproportionate early burden of the epidemic in sub-Saharan Africa was in the region around Lake Victoria, Africa's largest freshwater lake and the source of the River Nile. Many of the hardest hit locations in the 1980s and 1990s were in lakeside districts and provinces in Uganda (Rakai district), Tanzania (Mwanza and Bukoba provinces), and Kenya (Nyanza province), where the first cases of HIV/AIDS were reported. The epidemic then spread across Eastern Africa before proceeding to Southern Africa, which currently bears the heaviest burden.[42] Understanding the historical and current HIV epidemic dynamics in this setting may yield significant and fresh insight into settings where the HIV epidemic has now become endemic and seemingly impervious to HIV prevention efforts.

*Social and Ecological Setting*

The most dominant geographic feature of Nyanza province is Lake Victoria. The widespread dependence of many Africans on the ecological and natural environment for their livelihood (for food, for water, for income) both in this setting and in many other parts of the continent makes it an important, though often ignored, actor in accounts of HIV epidemics.[43] I will show how the environment was consequential in shaping young women's HIV risk in chapter 6.

I focused my fieldwork in four Nyanza province districts that border Lake Victoria: Bondo (north of the lake), Kisumu (central, and which includes the capital city), Nyando (central), and Homa Bay (south of the lake). Following the ratification of the constitution in 2010, Kenya adopted a county system, transforming 72 districts into 47 counties. With this system, these four districts are now subsumed under three counties: Siaya county (Bondo district), Kisumu county (Kisumu and Nyando districts), and Homa Bay county (Homa Bay district). These settings were selected to provide geographic diversity, while remaining in what is known as Luo-Nyanza.[44] The map on the following page illustrates the locations where the study was conducted.

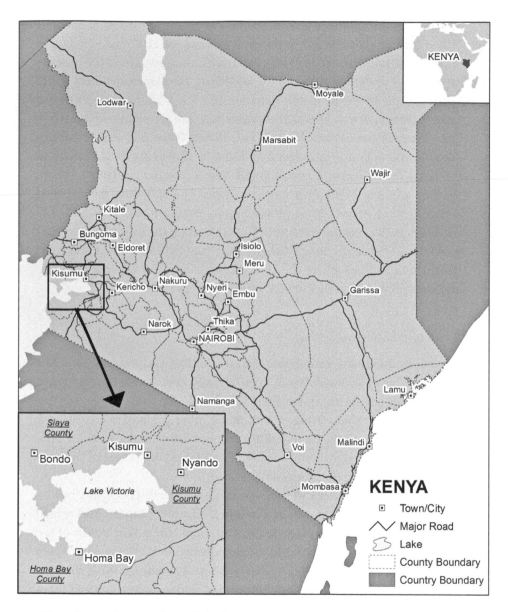

*Map.* Kenya. Cartographer: Elisabeth Root.

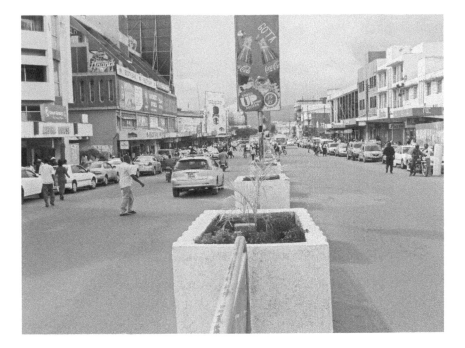

*Figure 5.* Downtown Kisumu city. Photograph by Jackson Wanga.

In the north, Bondo is characterized by rolling plains, sandy soils, grass-lands, hills, four islands, and 67 fish-landing beaches. Fishing is a major component of the district's local economy. Kisumu district, the location of the capital of the province and the nation's third-largest city, is south and east of Bondo district. It is a vibrant hub not just of the province, but indeed of the entire region; it lies not only on a major highway and railway line leading to Uganda and west and to South Sudan and north, but also, along with Uganda and Tanzania, on the banks of Lake Victoria. Thus, it serves as a major port city that facilitates trade between Kenya and the two other East African countries, and as a pass-through for trade from landlocked African countries to the coast of the Indian Ocean in southeast Kenya. Kisumu has about 50 miles of shoreline and 13 fish-landing beaches. Additionally, many factories and trading centers are based here. (See figure 5.)

To Kisumu's south and east lies Nyando. It is characterized by three distinct geographical features: the Nandi Hills, shared with the Kalenjin

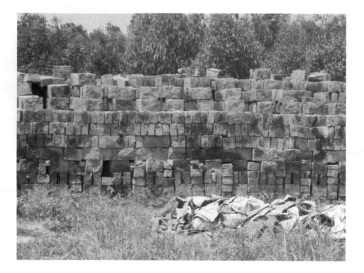

*Figure 6.* Brick making. Photograph by Jackson Wanga.

and Nandi peoples; Nyabondo Plateau; and the Kano plains. On the plateau, because of the bounty of natural stone, the key industries are brick and concrete making; on the plains, rice farming is an important industry. (See figure 6 and figure 7.)

Finally, on the far end of the lake, directly south and across the water from Bondo is Homa Bay. Its landscape is characterized by lowlands along the lakeshore and upland plateaus; it also has several beaches and small islands near its coastline. Distinctive features of Homa Bay are the humpbacked hills that line the landscape as one approaches the town as well as several rivers that crisscross the district.[45] (See figure 8.)

## STUDY METHODS

### Qualitative Fieldwork

My primary fieldwork was conducted between December 2005 and August 2006 and included 74 individual and focus group interviews among 185 youth (15–29 years old), middle-aged adults (35–55 years old),

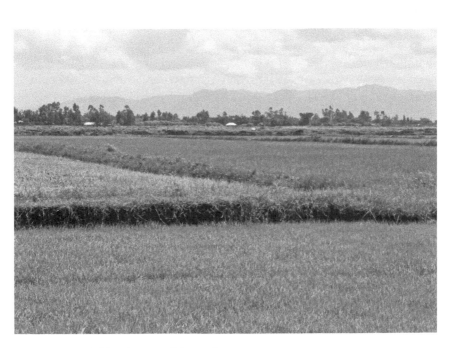

*Figure 7.* Rice fields. Photograph by Jackson Wanga.

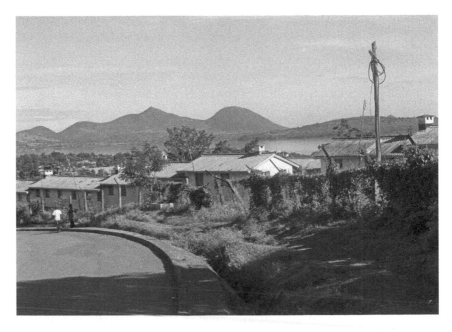

*Figure 8.* Homa Bay town. Photograph by Jackson Wanga.

and older adults (56–93 years old). Since then, I have returned at least once a year to the province, though not in a research capacity. To begin my study, I randomly selected 15 secondary (high) and vocational schools in the locations of interest in Nyanza province from the Kenya Education Directory, an annually updated, complete listing of all the schools in Kenya, and then proceeded to each one.[46] The schools were varying combinations of public and private, rural and urban, provincial and district, boarding and day. Rural schools often required a few hours of travel by road followed by several miles of walking. The experience of getting to these schools highlighted the physical isolation of many of them from even the nearest town, as well as the surprising reach of globalization and globalized messages of consumption, modernity, and HIV/AIDS. Selecting schools at random allowed for several starting points through which to conduct snowball sampling into different communities around the province. I conducted most community interviews in homes immediately surrounding the schools to capture young people who were not in school, as well as middle-aged adults and older adults. Additionally, respondents were recruited as individuals and in groups from community settings such as market places, villages, hospitals, community centers, and fish-landing beaches, and during social events where locals were gathered. Here I was reliant on friends of friends who served as local contacts, friendships and acquaintances developed in the course of my time in Nyanza, and the kind of boldness to simply start up conversations with strangers often required of field researchers. This approach allowed for data gathering from a combination of formal and noninstitutionalized settings. I also conducted interviews with 20 key informants, including government officials, local researchers, teachers, and community leaders. I asked study respondents about general issues facing the province (an icebreaker question initiating interviews), questions relating to young people's transitions to adulthood (about relationship formation, education, employment, and financial access), and questions about whether they felt HIV/AIDS was a problem in their community. Research material also included regularly written field notes documenting ethnographic observations and aspects of the culture and people's everyday lives not captured by formal taped interviews. The study protocol was approved by the University of Chicago's social sciences institutional review board, the Ministry of Education,

Republic of Kenya, and the Nyanza district and school officials overseeing the sites of study.

My two Luo research assistants were able guides and companions as I made my way through fieldwork: Marian, who had recently graduated high school, accompanied and assisted me during most of my fieldwork; and Rose, who had a master's in sociology, provided assistance in the final month of fieldwork while Marian transitioned to university to pursue her bachelor's degree in education. I benefited from many interesting conversations with them over the months of fieldwork as we talked about what we had seen or heard in our travels. Conversations with Marian, who was a peer in many ways of those I was interviewing, were especially beneficial. She corrected some of my assumptions, and noted things about different settings that, as a nonlocal, I would not have noticed. For example, we realized that we had different ways of assessing whether a household was wealthy when, after an interview in a hut, she noted that the household was relatively wealthy because they had a cow in the yard, unlike other households in the area.

Interviews were conducted in English and Kiswahili (the national languages), which, as a Kenyan native, I was fluent in, as well as in dhoLuo, the local ethnic group language, which I learned in the course of fieldwork. Along with Marian and Rose, I transcribed taped interviews and, where needed, translated them into English. I then conducted all coding and analyses of interview transcripts and field notes recording ethnographic observations. Both my data collection and analysis were guided by grounded theory; emergent themes and theories from early parts of the fieldwork shaped subsequent interviews, and a variety of interview themes were pursued until data and theoretical saturation was reached.[47] In the chapters to follow, where respondents spoke in English, I try as much as possible to preserve their original phrasings and grammar to avoid making them sound like they speak Queen's English, and I provide explanation or clarification where needed. All names of respondents and schools are pseudonyms to preserve privacy and anonymity.[48] For the same reason, because towns and villages are small and because many settings were characterized by thick social networks of friends, relatives, and acquaintances (as I quickly came to realize), I do not explicitly name the specific locations I visited.

## Survey Data

I complemented qualitative fieldwork with quantitative survey analysis using data from the 2003 and 2008–9 Kenya Demographic and Health Surveys (KDHS 2004 and KDHS 2010). The KDHS surveys are nationally representative, household-based surveys of women (15–49) and men (15–54) that have been conducted every five years since 1989. The last two surveys, in 2003 and 2008–9, included HIV testing, with fairly high response rates for men and women.[49] All statistical analyses in this book are based on those who were tested for HIV. I draw on KDHS 2004 for historical trends especially in chapter 3, and on KDHS 2010 for contemporary trends throughout the rest of the book. While the survey data are robust for estimating national trends and carrying out statistical analyses on the national data, a key limitation in their use for this study is the small sample sizes of Luo-Nyanza respondents (respondents of Luo ethnicity residing in Nyanza province), which limit similar group-specific analyses. Because of this limitation, my primary use of the data for the Luo-Nyanza population in this book is descriptive, presenting population-weighted trends of a variety of factors such as HIV prevalence, education, and employment. I also provide sample sizes and confidence intervals of these estimates in the appendix.

## Mixing Methods

Grounded theory also shaped my back-and-forth movement between survey and fieldwork data, both during data collection and in subsequent data analysis and writing. Emergent codes in the qualitative material were explored in the quantitative data and vice versa. For example, the gender disparity in HIV rates in the survey among Luo-Nyanza youth prompted focus groups and individual interviews that concentrated on young men's relationships with same-aged partners (or lack thereof as it turned out, which is discussed in chapter 4). Interview reports of an increasing number of relationships of men just out of school prompted closer survey analysis of how young men's HIV rates increased each year as they approached their late 20s. And, the nonlinear nature of the link between educational attainment and HIV rates revealed in survey analysis provoked a deeper qualitative exploration of what was going on in school (chapter 5).

My main assumption in using this kind of mixed-method analysis was that, while appreciating that different logics of inquiry underlie the interviews driven by structured categories that produce survey data and the unstructured fieldwork that allows categories to emerge, they are nonetheless accessing different aspects of the *same* social reality inhabited by the people of Luo-Nyanza. In particular, characterizing and understanding the HIV risk environment in which young people were navigating their relationships required attention to three things: the numbers (for example, who was infected, by how much); the lived experiences of those embodying those numbers (for example, the logics guiding relationship decision-making); and the social-structural processes both producing those numbers and shaping those lived experiences, especially in institutional contexts such as schools and labor markets, which involve so many young people.

## REFLEXIVITY AND THE MARGINAL WOMAN

For much of my fieldwork, though I traveled and stayed in different areas throughout the province for varying lengths of time, my primary base was in Maseno, a small town in Kisumu district, located 40 minutes away from the province capital, Kisumu. I stayed with paternal relatives who lived near the main road. With easy access to public transport, fairly reliable electricity, and space to write, their place was ideal for my work. In several senses, I was Robert Park's "marginal (wo)man," belonging, yet not quite belonging, understanding, yet not quite understanding. I was familiar with the mud-floor houses and kitchens, the corrugated iron and thatched roofs, walking through the hills on narrow pathways, the slower pace of life, timing my travel to avoid torrential downpours, negotiating public transport, and the endless waiting for public officials. There was no learning or assimilating there. I was unfamiliar with much else: the language spoken by the ethnic group (which I had to learn), the daily mundane logics underlying how the Luo people lived life and approached situations, and the varying ways in which I was perceived as I traveled throughout the province. I engaged in participant observation and took regular field notes. I talked with local informants, getting to know them and learning their world through the words they said, the things they did, and the places they took me. I wrote field notes on everything I saw, from my daily transportation experiences, to descriptions of the landscape, my own feelings about particular places and people, events that took place, and so on. I talked to many people I encountered, such as a lady on the beach selling fish and the bike-taxi men who transported me long distances to schools and other locations. In community interviews, I was highly dependent on informant networks—who they knew and which groups they could convene at short notice.

Fieldwork was characterized by many moments of mutual recognition and strangeness. I was perceived as a strange anomaly in a context where many young women drop out of school to get married, since I was an unmarried, childless young Kenyan woman studying for a PhD in America, the land of many people's dreams. But I looked like them, sometimes sounded like them, dressed like them, and shared their nationality and heritage. Yet perhaps the most powerful personal moments of recognition throughout fieldwork and after were when I observed the similarities between the consuming young women who are the subjects of this book and those I observed while I was writing and later teaching as a graduate student at the University of Chicago and then as an assistant professor at the University of Colorado in Boulder, several thousand miles—but not worlds—away. It was just that, in Africa, young women's lives were more likely to end in tragedy. Far from an impersonal and purely academic account, then, this book is a study about the young women whose dangerous transitions I might have had to traverse except for the strange turns my life has taken.

Chapter 2 examines the widespread nature of transactional sex relationships, both in Africa as well as the United States. Specifically, the chapter illustrates the centrality of consumption to intimate partnerships in both settings, explores how consuming women are cultivated and produced, and examines similarities in the gendered entanglement of love, money, and consumption among women in vastly different places and historical time periods. In doing so, I show not only why women living in the wealthiest African households have the highest rates of HIV, but also how this entanglement places young African women at disproportionate risk for acquiring HIV.

Chapter 3 begins with a discussion of the density of death that resulted from living in a high HIV-prevalence environment, and how the Luo of Nyanza province navigated this social reality. I then describe the study's historical and cultural context to set the context for the contemporary transitions to adulthood that are explored in subsequent chapters. Specifically, I describe how young people in this setting historically came of age, their relationship-formation processes, the changing socioeconomy among the Luo ethnic group over the twentieth century, and consequent shifts in attitudes toward mass education, salaried employment, and norms of beauty, money, and consumption.

In chapter 4, I show how intimate relationships and communities enable and motivate girls' transformation into consuming women. The chapter examines how Luo youth characterized their relationships (for example, "relationships for sex" and "relationships for education"), how they initiated relationships and found partners, and their motivations underlying partner selection. I connect these choices to the HIV trends, showing the epidemiological riskiness of young women's partnerships. Specifically, I show how these characterizations and motivations combined to make the selection of "safe" same-aged partners relatively less attractive (at least in the short term) than the selection of "dangerous" older partners. I show how money came to be central to intimate-relationship formation, and I link this to historical changes in the socioeconomy, ideals of beauty, and consumption practices documented in chapter 3. Finally, I explore the implications of relationship logics in this setting in relation to key HIV-prevention strategies (abstinence, condom use, faithfulness, and HIV testing).

Chapter 5 shows how girls are produced as consuming women in the institutional context of school by exploring the complicated role of school in young women's lives. I show how schools, charged with constructing modern subjects, also contribute to the construction of gendered processes that place young women at risk. I begin with a discussion of the paradox of educated women's HIV risk and the nonlinear relationship between education and HIV. I then describe the rise of mass education in Africa, and Kenya in particular, before discussing the contemporary pursuit of education, including the rising constraints to access, associated expenses, and subsequent disillusionment. The rest of the chapter explores how school complicates young women's attempts to stay HIV free.

Specifically, I explore the gendered construction of "needs" and its ties to consumption and modernity. I show how social-structural processes in school (for example, peer groups and the structure of the school calendar) both entrench these constructions and inadvertently facilitate transactional relationships, even while ostensibly seeking to regulate schoolgirl behavior. I discuss the dueling normative systems girls are choosing among, one urging them to wait to consume, and the other urging them to combine consumption and relationships with education. I conclude the chapter with case studies of young women's pursuit of education, as well as with reflections on the implications of the chapter findings for school-going girls in other African settings.

In chapter 6, I explore how gendered labor markets exacerbate the challenges young women face once they leave school, having been produced as consuming subjects. I describe their experiences as they confront a challenging economic environment in which their great needs meet limited means. I describe the kinds of jobs young women take up, the disillusionment faced in dealing with unemployment and itinerant work, and the reduction in financial support from parents and guardians on leaving school. In particular, I show how youth transitioning out of school confront a gendered labor market, gendered in access to jobs and in types of jobs and, as a result, gendered in access to and amount of income. I show how this is consequential for relationship formation and HIV risk for young women, and why women who work are at particular risk for HIV. In the second part of the chapter, I bring together many of the themes discussed in this book by engaging in a close study of fishing, a major lucrative industry in this area. I explore how the ecostructural context of Lake Victoria mapped onto the gendered fishing economy and combined to shape young women's relationships with fishermen and their HIV risk. Specifically, I illustrate how environmental changes in Lake Victoria and the surrounding area conditioned the sexual relationships and sexual mixing patterns of fisherfolk and young women. I show how this was exacerbated by a gendered fishing economy where only men fished and had access to daily income, in contrast to many locals in surrounding lakeside communities who lived on less than a dollar a day.

In the final chapter of the book, I propose a gendered and life-course perspective to HIV prevention, and apply the findings from this book to a consideration of individual, institutional, and ecostructural HIV-prevention strategies that might be usefully combined to reduce young African women's HIV risk, both among the Luo and in other parts of Africa.

The epilogue reflects on the current push to scale up antiretroviral therapy across sub-Saharan Africa, and considers both its promise and its limits in preventing HIV among young African women.

## 2 Consuming Women, Modernity, and HIV Risk

You know, if you are a schoolgirl, it is very hard to get
money unless you are given by your parent, and let's say
there is a very nice trouser you want to buy and you cannot
ask your father or mother for money. Now it will force you
to look for a boyfriend whose parents are a bit rich so that if
you beg for something like Kshs 1000 [$14.28], he can eas-
ily give you so that you can go and buy that trouser that you
are really in need of, but if, let's say, you are working in
somebody's house, it will force you to scrub that house
every morning but at the end of the month, you only earn
100 shillings. [So] if you have a boyfriend, you can earn it
very easily because you only go there, do it once, then he
gives you.

Jacqueline, high school girl

In this chapter, I will show how consumption has become an integral part
of what it means to be a modern woman, and situate this identity transformation within the linked sites of gendered and sexual economies that
many young women inhabit. I pay particular attention to transactional sex
relationships, and show how they are a product of the entanglement of
love and money not just in relationships across Africa, but also in the
United States, both historically and in contemporary times. In doing this,
I will show how the entwinement of intimacy and money is not unique to
Africa; rather, its occurrence there is merely illustrative of *globalized*
gendered dynamics in many parts of the world where the marketing and

promotion of the consumption of goods work to make modernity and romance synonymous with consumption. I will use historical and contemporary examples of these dynamics in different parts of Africa as well as in the United States to illustrate these similarities.

Making these comparisons across a variety of sociopolitical and historical settings, and drawing on and juxtaposing both Western and Africanist scholars may sometimes appear jarring; this is intentional. The historical norm has been to assume difference, and even sometimes extreme difference, between Western sexualities and African sexualities and their shaping both on the continent and in the diaspora. The effect has been to exoticize and treat Africa and its sexualities as "other."[1] The aim of this chapter is to do the opposite.

In addition to historicizing transactional relationships, I also deexoticize them by highlighting the *similarities* between gendered entanglements of love, money, and consumption among women in different settings, and discuss how these entanglements have been cultivated and co-opted by marketing companies in similar ways among women in the United States and various African settings. I will provide several empirical examples to allow readers to see these similarities for themselves. In doing this, I will show that transactional sex is not unique to African settings when we really think about what it is and how it works. Indeed, by examining what is and has happened "at home" in the United States in this chapter before exploring these dynamics among the Luo of Kenya in subsequent chapters, I challenge Western readers to rethink a context with which they are familiar. By making "familiar" relationships in the United States "strange," my hope is that the seemingly "strange" relationships of young African women across the continent and among the Luo in particular in this and subsequent chapters will start to seem familiar.

What might also be jarring for scholars as they read this and subsequent chapters is my taking not just urban but also rural spaces in Africa seriously as a space in which globalized processes unfold—in particular, my asserting similarities between consuming young women in rural settings in Kenya and consuming young women in the United States with radical differences in their economic location by juxtaposing examples and scholars writing about both settings. James Ferguson has argued that Africa is often an "inconvenient case" for globalization scholars, barely addressed, if at all, because of its continued and indeed exacerbated poverty and because of its seeming isolation from global flows of capital, consumption, and direct investment. Indeed, it has often provided an example of modernity in reverse, with its best days lying in the past, economically as well as in terms of, for example, life expectancy. However, what these scholars have missed, he notes, is just how extensively drawn in sub-Saharan Africa is and has been to the global economy. It simply requires, he argues, a recharacterization of what globalization looks like on the ground in Africa. Rather than thinking about globalization as a phenomena best captured by studying the extent of global flows with widespread coverage in a setting, Africa provides examples of extensive point-to-point connectivity across global spaces, between enclaves of resource extraction such as mining and oil sites, numerous international nongovernmental organizations with multiple branches across the continent, the middle class and elites in several African cities, global finance institutions, multinational corporations and donors, and African-born diaspora in cities across Europe and North America. And even then, Africa's rural and poorest cannot and should not be excluded. Employees at these sites and organizations and members of the middle class and elite have deep and extensive ties to the poor, ties through which portions of the global flow. Additionally, "modern" consumption is available used and at a deep discount—through secondhand North Face clothing that has made its way from Western charities, for example, or through cheap pay-as-you-go Nokia mobile phones. As the Comaroffs put it, "modernity has always been both one thing and many, always both a universal project and a host of specific parochial emplacements, a force for equality and simultaneously a producer of difference." Thus, how modernity is done and produced will look *both* similar and different depending on a reader's social location; its story is about both one kind of modernity and many alternative modernities.[2] There is both something global, familiar, and even taken for granted (as I illustrate in this chapter) and something local, strange, and startling (as I illustrate in specific detail in subsequent chapters) about how modernity, consumption, gendered disparities in HIV rates, and the role of transactional relationships in producing them are linked together. In this next section, I first begin with discussing transactional relationships in Africa, before discussing them as they unfold in the United States.

## TRANSACTIONAL SEX RELATIONSHIPS IN AFRICA

Perhaps the most striking similarity in qualitative accounts of young African women's higher HIV risk across the continent is what has been termed "transactional sex relationships"—noncommercial, nonmarital sexual relationships involving the exchange of money and gifts. These relationships have been documented among young women in settings ranging from Ghana, Nigeria, Senegal, and Cameroon in West Africa, to Botswana and South Africa in Southern Africa, to Kenya, Uganda, Madagascar, and Malawi in Eastern Africa, to name a few.[3] While many of these relationships involve only two participants at a given time (serial monogamy), some of the examples documented in the literature are of women at the more extreme end of number of concurrent partnerships maintained. For example, Francis Nyamnjoh described some young West African college women who maintained three partners—one they love (*le chic*), one to help financially (*le cheque*), and one to help with school work (*le choc*)—to enable them to achieve the four Vs—"*villa, voiture, voyages, virement bancaire*" (house, car, travel, and bank transfers). Jennifer Cole described young Malagasy women who maintained two partners—a *jaombilo* (a similar-aged unemployed boyfriend) they love and keep, and a *vazaha* (an older European gentleman) who supports them financially. In South Africa, Mark Hunter gave an example of a young woman who was asked what each of her three partners gave her. She responded, "one money . . . another Checkers groceries . . . another buys me clothes."[4] The men profiled are often slightly older (two to three years) or much older (over 10 years) working men. Unfortunately, older men have higher rates of HIV, and a young woman's partnerships with one or more older partners who provide increase her probability of encountering an HIV-positive partner. Transactional relationships are characterized as problematic precisely because, as long as money and gifts are central motivations for the relationship, young women may engage in concurrent partnerships to maximize the amount they receive from men, thus increasing their HIV risk. Further, wealthy men have a greater ability to maintain multiple partners, thus simultaneously placing many women at risk if they are HIV positive; in addition, economically dependent young women may have reduced leverage to negotiate safe sex.[5]

Accounts of young women's transactional relationships are especially striking because they are rarely about "survival sex," that is, sexual relationships to receive money to buy basics such as food. Neither are they usually about "commercial sex," the explicit exchange of sex for money, where sex is a job women engage in for their livelihood. Indeed, the women profiled are more often women who are not destitute, and many are school- or college-going young women. This is at least partly supported by the fact that women living in the wealthiest households in Africa have higher rates of HIV than the poorest women.[6] (The same is also true for men.)[7] In the surveys on which this finding is based, wealth is a measure of a household's ownership of consumer goods such as household effects (clocks, radios, televisions, mobile and landline phones, fridges, solar panels), means of transportation (bicycles, cars, motorbikes, boats), land and home ownership, water access, and toilet facilities.[8] To a large extent, the measure is an index of how drawn in to the modern consumer economy a given household is. In Kenya, women living in the poorest households by this measure have the *lowest* rates of HIV, and those living in the richest households have the *highest* rates of HIV. Among young women (under 30), those living in middle-wealth households have the highest rates of HIV.[9]

Thus, to the extent that transactional relationships underlie young women's higher HIV rates, it is not the poorest women engaging in them, but women who are fairly well off to begin with. Young women's transactional relationships, then, are less about survival or livelihood. They are about, as Suzanne Leclerc-Madlala argues, the pursuit of modernity.[10] The dominant signifier of modernity for many young women is the purchase, consumption, and display of modern goods. Indeed, there is a sense in reading these accounts that transactional relationships as a means for enhanced consumption are an indelible part of the landscape of young African women's relationships. Unlike commercial sex relationships, however, this receipt of money and gifts is *embedded* within intimate, sometimes romantic and loving relationships. Participants are not "patron" and "client"; they are "boyfriend" and "girlfriend."[11] In other words, even while the desire for money and gifts is among the expectations in such relationships, issues of love and trust are often also considered at stake.[12]

The widespread documentation of monetary or gift giving in the context of sexual relationships across sub-Saharan Africa does not mean that every young woman engages in such relationships. However, an extensive review of the literature on transactional relationships suggested that "in general, the findings point to large majorities of adolescent girls who have been involved in transactional sexual relations."[13] In Kisumu, Nyanza, for example, three-quarters of men surveyed reported giving an average of 10% of their monthly income to their nonmarital, noncommercial sexual partners.[14] This level suggests that transaction in intimate relationships was the *norm* rather than the exception in this setting.

In some ways, then, to mark out these kinds of sexual relationships in which (predominantly one-way, male-to-female) money or gift giving occurs as "transactional" is something of a misnomer. As Hunter noted, "sex, like all embodied practices, is always simultaneously material and meaningful in complex ways."[15] Marriage, the principal intimate relationship in the eyes of many states and societies, is as much financial as it is romantic and companionate. Indeed, marriage as a desired end of the dating and courtship process is, in many ways, the ultimate and culminating "transactional relationship," and as Adam Ashforth noted of young unemployed South African men's dilemma, "the road to marriage is paved with money."[16]

## TRANSACTIONAL RELATIONSHIPS IN THE UNITED STATES

The practice of men's money serving as the basis of dating and courtship practices is true not just in Africa but also in the West. Beth Bailey, for example, documented the historical shift in the United States away from calling practices in the 1920s, where men would call at the residence of their desired partner and the lady and her family would be responsible for the at-home entertainment. The rise of dating in subsequent decades, however, shifted courtship "from the front porch to the back seat." Increasingly, dates were conducted in public spheres such as restaurants and diners, movie theatres, and dance halls. All these venues, along with a car to transport the man and his date to them (and provide private space for physical intimacy), required money, and specifically men's money. The complaints by young American men unable to pay were documented in a variety of sources such as "letters to the editor" in various newspapers. The main message from them seems to be an almost universal complaint among young men caught in the same social-structural trap. Decades later and an ocean away, young Ugandan university men's frustration was encapsulated in the title of an article, "No Romance without Finance,"[17] and young Kenyan men in this current study bitterly noted to me, "no money, no room for you."

Eva Ilouz documents the increasing embeddedness of contemporary Western consumption in dating, such that romance without any form of consumption has come to seem incomplete. Sending flowers, a box of chocolates, a honeymoon in an exotic location have become synonymous with romance,[18] with an invisible and assumed male provision and facilitation of it. Even if a couple today splits costs down the middle—going Dutch—in Western contexts during dating and courtship, there is frequently still the surprisingly intransigent expectation that a man will spend large sums of money on certain big-ticket items such as engagement rings. While the gendered disparities in access to money and resources, and the kinds of expenditures men incur, clearly vary dramatically across global settings, it remains striking that the flow of resources seems generally greater from men to women than vice versa.

Contemporary Western ideologies and rhetoric around "pure" romance make it anathema to discuss love and money in the same breath. This "hostile worlds" approach described by Viviana Zelizer assumes that "such a profound contradiction exists between intimate social relations and monetary transfers that any contact between the two spheres inevitably leads to moral contamination and degradation"—hence, the reference to women who sell sex as "prostitutes."[19] The exchange of money turns the sex into a commodity, and the women providing this commodity are morally condemned. However, as she demonstrates both historically and in the eyes of the law, intimate relationships are inextricably intertwined with monetary transfers. Relationships have "differentiated ties . . . each marked by a distinctive pattern of payment. . . . People adopt symbols, rituals, practices, and physically distinguishable forms of money to mark distinct social relations."[20] Thus, the timing of the cash exchange, immediately before or after sex, would be the distinguishing feature for commercial sex;[21] cash exchanges at times seemingly unassociated with when sex takes place would suggest other kinds of relationships. Similarly, we might observe different monetary and gift-giving practices distinguishing dating, cohabiting, engagement, the wedding, and marriage itself. What is striking is the extent to which consumption has become *symbolic* of love.

Thinking about diamond engagement rings is a case in point. For example, bigger and more expensive diamond rings on newly engaged women's fingers often elicit comments from friends, family, and strangers alike about how much the man loves the woman, implicitly suggesting that the size of the ring is the ultimate expression of the magnitude of his love. The constant jewelry advertisements targeted at men during the peak engagement season between Christmas and Valentine's Day are geared toward making potential male consumers believe that "love needs to be nourished and should be constantly cultivated through consumption." Jewelry thus becomes "codified love."[22] This association between love and consumption is no accident, and is, in fact, explicitly cultivated by marketers. Love—as well as the romance purported to nourish it—is a highly profitable motivation for (continual) consumption. N.W. Ayer, a famous American advertiser, made the following recommendation in 1938 at the onset of a massive US campaign to make diamond rings ubiquitous: "Since young men buy over 90% of all engagement rings, it would be crucial to *inculcate* in them the idea that diamonds [are] a gift of love: the larger and finer the diamond, the greater the expression of love. Similarly, young women ha[ve] to be encouraged to view diamonds as an *integral* part of any romantic courtship. [We need] to make it a *psychological necessity* capable of competing successfully at the retail level with utility goods and services" (my emphasis).[23]

The campaign was apparently a success. An article in 2007 declared that more than 80% of American brides had love expressed to them through receiving an engagement ring, at an average cost of $3200 in 2006.[24] A survey in 2011 by the top two wedding websites in the United States found that the cost had risen to $5200, despite the tough recession.[25]

Gifts in and of themselves, especially in the context of romantic relationships, would be considered unproblematic except for that fact that, as many analysts acknowledge, they carry sometimes significant social obligations to reciprocate.[26] Gifts are not "free." Beth Bailey noted how young women struggled with holding the line on how much physical intimacy to allow as recipients of their partner's financial largess in a climate where premarital pregnancy was highly stigmatized and where they were cast as gatekeepers of their sexual virtue. Transaction, then, is also problematic insofar as young women's choices about reciprocity are constrained. That is, it is difficult to say no to sex for an extended period of time to a man who has been continually generous and who has thus continually demonstrated "love."

## HISTORICAL UNDERPINNINGS OF GENDERED, GENERATIONAL, AND SEXUAL ECONOMIES

Transactional sex relationships do not occur in a social-structural ahistorical vacuum; these sexual economies, fueled in part by monetary transactions, are structured by *gendered* access to money and resources with long historical underpinnings. In other words, the predominantly one-way flow of money and resources—from men to women—is illustrative of the fact that capital and labor markets have historically been and still are gendered, as I will illustrate in this and subsequent chapters. That is, in even the most advanced countries, despite radical changes during the twentieth and early twenty-first century, men make more money than women. This is because they are more likely to inherit or create wealth, and they are paid more than women.

This phenomenon is no less true in sub-Saharan Africa, where a key historical antecedent was colonizers across the subcontinent setting in place gendered economies to control local populations and maximize resource extraction. The labor-migration system set up during the colonial era in many Central, East, and Southern African countries resulted in urban towns, mining areas, and other such work sites being dominated by working men, with access to limited wage income; meanwhile, villages, or "reserves," were dominated by financially dependent women, periodically visited (annually or every 18 months) by their men, as colonizers allowed.[27] In Nairobi, Kenya's capital, for example, the historian Luise White documented how men, unable to bring their families to live with them in the city, sought the few resident city women for "the comforts of home." Eluding an easy classification as commercial sex workers, these women, along with providing sexual services, also cooked, cleaned, and cared for these men. It was essentially the classic marital bargain—male financial provision in exchange for female domestic and sexual provision—without the formal title of "wife." Outside of these "jobs," women had limited avenues for supporting themselves in the city. Indeed, in some cases, young women left rural families to go to the city temporarily to earn money in this way before returning home to respectability and marriage. James Ferguson documented how Zambian women were classified as "wives" by male miners in order to gain access to "family housing" in the mining compounds. Men provided housing and other financial support to women with whom they were having sexual relationships, but to whom they were not necessarily married or in serious relationships. Without male support, women would not have the financial means to live in the city. Indeed, women's ability to live independently outside of marriage or an intimate sexual relationship with a man was structurally severely limited, making it difficult for them to survive without a man's support.[28] This situation continues to represent the contemporary reality for the many African women who earn less than men and the many for whom access to land for subsistence farming (especially for those engaged in the nonwage labor force) and a home is structurally dependent on providing men such as fathers and husbands.[29]

Marriage as a primary means of economic security and social mobility for women is not unique to African settings. In the United States, historically, men's legally higher pay was justified as a "breadwinner" wage, structured to take into account the wife and children a man was supporting; women's lower pay was thus seen as providing a useful supplement to a husband's or father's income.[30] Even though laws have since changed, making such wage discrimination illegal, recent studies on gender wage inequality in the United States show the persistence of these beliefs reflected in differential pay for mothers and fathers, even in an advanced twenty-first-century economy. While married fathers enjoy a wage premium—a "daddy bonus"—married mothers experience a "motherhood penalty" earning 4% less per child they have.[31]

Structured access to money and resources is not only gendered, but also often *generational*. Examining briefly practices of bride-wealth exchange in Africa—a primary way in which capital has circulated and in several cases still circulates—provides a particularly useful way of illustrating this dimension. Bride-wealth exchange (in contrast to dowry) occurs when money and gifts are given by the groom's family to the bride's family to contract a marriage. It was and is practiced in several patrilineal African societies, including the most dominant ethnic group in Nyanza, the Luo.[32] Bride wealth underscores the idea not only that women were being exchanged between households[33]—from the household of one man to the household of another man—but also that this was the means through which *wealth* from the household of one man moved to the household of another man. The exchange of wealth (money, animals, food, and other gifts) between previously unrelated households was always embedded in intimate relationships between men and women, particularly when they were still fragile and in formation. This exchange was also structured by generation, whereby a young woman's marriage provided the opportunity for an older man from one household to acquire wealth from another older man's household.[34]

Transactional sex relationships in Africa are a contemporary, gendered, and generational subversion of this tradition. In an economic context, where many men can no longer afford formal bride wealth,[35] smaller transactions are made, not between two men, but from an older or slightly older man to a younger woman. In this way, young women gain access to money and resources that might usually have gone predominantly to fathers and male relatives. Indeed, when access to money and resources is structurally constrained, transactional sex emerges as a way of "redistribution and reciprocity in an unequal and uncertain world," where men's dominant access to wealth and resources "compels them" to have concurrent sexual partnerships involving transactional sex.[36] These men with relative wealth are not necessarily much older men; rather, they are men who are working—"working-class men"—and whose transfers, though monetarily small in absolute terms, represent sizable proportions of their income.

Perhaps what is really underlying anxiety about transactional sex relationships is that money—decoupled from marriage—is being redirected to young women, a group of people usually disenfranchised with limited access to power and resources. That is, money and gifts women receive are not necessarily directed toward families and communities in the manner of bride wealth, but rather are used for the individualized, short-term consumption of modern goods. Transactional relationships disrupt long-term flows of wealth that serve to uphold social-structural[37] and patriarchal reproduction in order to serve shorter-term ends—conspicuous noncommunal consumption by young women. (I discuss some of these anxieties in chapter 3.) This also highlights the role that marriage—as a declared or purported end goal in a relationship—serves as a *legitimating* lens through which entanglements of love and money are viewed. Thus, receiving thousands of dollars in the form of a diamond ring from one's fiancé is socially sanctioned in ways that a similar receipt from someone with whom one has just "hooked up" and does not plan to see again is not.

Why, however, are transactional relationships in Africa persisting amid an HIV pandemic? To the extent that young African women have agency in the entering and exiting of relationships, as many accounts document that they do, why do they continually place themselves in these relationships? If consumption is driving these relationships, why do young women feel compelled to consume?

## CONSUMING WOMEN

As readers looking into the world of young African women with desires for consumption far above their own ability to afford it in the chapters to follow, it might be hard not to share the same gendered moral anxiety: disapproving of consumption not related to survival, young women having these desires rather than young men, and the compounding of the situation when sexual relationships are involved.[38] Yet focusing solely on young women's choices blinds us not only to the gendered and generational economic imbalance in access to resources to meet those desires (as I briefly discussed earlier), but also to the explicit and gendered cultivation of consumer desires. Indeed, consuming women have been and are *produced* in similar ways across varied contexts.

Consumption was and has been understood as feminine, especially in the West.[39] As Friedman noted, "Since Western nations began building consumer economies, the consuming woman has been constituted as an object of dread and ridicule, fear and desire, a figure whose wants and needs some seek to suppress, others to incite."[40] A primary way in which women were produced as consumers was by framing consumer goods as *necessities* for a variety of ends. In other words, these wants and needs were not "natural" to womanhood; they were cultivated. Women were cultivated in this way not just in Western nations, but also in African ones. Timothy Burke, for example, notes in his study of consumption in Zimbabwe:

> Just as educators and missionaries had held women as responsible for transforming the social content of African life—accepting in their own way the dictum that the personal is political—marketers believed fervently that women were the key to changing the material composition of the African home, that women controlled most purchases and most tastes. Of course, many of the "soft" nondurable consumer goods, especially toiletries, that made up the bulk of business in the "African market" were primarily considered to be *for* women or to lie *within* their appointed domestic sphere. In general, however, women were pegged as somehow holding the key to the successful creation and reproduction of *new needs*.[41]

His book illustrates how needs for toiletries, soaps, perfumes, and other such products became seen as necessities in colonial Zimbabwe by showing, for example, explicit ways in which marketers for products manufactured by firms such as the Lever brothers (who later merged with another company to form Unilever) and Colgate-Palmolive sought to cultivate "problems" and solutions or "new needs" requiring the consumption of advertised products in mid-twentieth-century Zimbabwe. African women were positioned and created as consumers, and then targeted as key to the consumption of domestic products, constituting a lucrative new market. There was more than consumption going on, however. In a colonial and racially segregated context, by consuming these products constructed as "needs," they were also buying *modernity,* Westernized (read "white") sophistication, smartness, class, and status mobility—attributes used heavily in the advertising and marketing of these products.

Similar dynamics were at work in the mid-twentieth-century United States, where a gendered separation of spheres reigned: the work sphere for men, the domestic sphere for women. Men were tasked as breadwinners primarily responsible for financial provision for the family, while women were primarily responsible for the care of the home and children.[42] The household, in similar ways to Zimbabwe, became a marketer's dream, with women targeted as potential consumers of labor-saving devices and other household goods. Women's consumption simultaneously was a key underpinning of department store and retail economies, which were booming in postwar America, and was yet subject to the anxious and morally disapproving fathers and husbands who had to fund them.[43] Women would be torn between expectations that they should be prudent housekeepers, frugal with their husband's money, and their being cultivated to be conscious of fashion, appliances, and household decor even before they got married. An excerpt from a *Ladies' Home Journal* from 1955 targeted at single women, which Bailey quotes, is illustrative of this:

> And I'm going to tell you a secret now. It's about girls and how they dress and how they do their hair. Men always think these things are frivolous matters. Nothing could be further from the truth. The girl in the red dress with the plunging neckline may only be shopping for a washing machine as she tangos so sensually upon the dance floor. She may know very well that it takes this dress to get that fellow to let her wash those clothes in that washing machine he's going to buy her when they are married.[44]

In other words, women were urged to look forward to the ability to consume their husband's discretionary income[45] in the purchase of new cutting-edge labor-saving devices that were the product of scientific and technological innovation—the very essence of modernity.

The construction of women as critical consumers in markets in Zimbabwe and in the United States was part of a broader globalized production of women who consumed to purchase modernity. In their study of the emergence of the "Modern Girl" among young women in the early to mid-twentieth century in Africa, Asia, Europe, and North America, whose "near simultaneous emergence was tied to the international circulation of commodity cultures, mass media and political discourse,"[46] the Modern Girl research group noted: "Early on, The Modern Girl research group recognized that a particular bundle of commodities including lipstick, nail polish, face creams and powders, skin lighteners, tanning lotions, shampoos, hair-styling products, fancy soaps, perfumes, deodorants, toothpastes, cigarettes, high-heeled shoes, cloche hats and fashionable, sexy clothes was advertised globally. We also realized that such commodities were linked in each local context to the expression of modern femininity."[47]

Young women in diverse settings and cities across the globe who were subject to localized versions of the "Modern Girl" in advertisements could *do modernity* through the consumption of these commodities. In South Africa in the 1930s, for example, there was a transformation from "traditional" to "modern" forms of beautification, as Lynn Thomas describes: "Xhosa-speaking young men and women used animal fat, butter, and by this period Vaseline to make their skin shine. They also enhanced their beauty through facial tattooing, washing daily, plaiting and applying red ochre to their hair, wearing sweet smelling leaves, and using love medicines. As school-educated Christians abandoned some of these practices, they adopted beauty and hygienic regimes involving store bought soaps and creams and the wearing of 'smart' clothing."[48]

Facilitated by mission schools and young South African women's training there in new domestic practices and routines in household management, participating in consumption was a marker of transformation. Commenting on the dynamics at a major Black magazine, Thomas notes that "what ongoing *Bantu World* discussions about the Modern Girl make clear is that the emergence of a group of school-educated young women committed to racial betterment could not be disentangled from the cultivation of new looks and consumptive practices."[49]

Against a backdrop of racial apartheid, young women's consumption was as much about doing modernity and class as it was, she argues, about racial respectability. Strikingly, Modern Girls around the world, through engaging in the same consumptive practices, looked the same in all respects except for skin color, whose difference skin-lightening creams and tanning lotions also sought to erase.

Single women also consumed to make themselves better marriage candidates. As noted earlier, consumption in the United States was central to dating practices. However, its role was no longer confined to young men's expenditures on women during dates and outings; young women spent to make themselves attractive marriage mates, especially when they perceived a scarcity of marriageable men. Young American women's dating lives were shaped by two key events: the Great Depression (1929–33) and World War II (1939–45). Perceived scarcity in the Depression was due to the fact that fewer young men could afford to marry. Women dated many different men before settling on one to marry. By World War II, however, the American economy was revitalized by war and there was unprecedented economic growth. The war contributed, in real terms, to a scarcity of men.[50] On the return of veterans, however, the GI Bill contributed to making them particularly eligible bachelors, with their entitlement to government provision of low-interest mortgage loans and subsidies for college and job training, among other benefits.[51] The shoe was on the other foot, and it was men who had their pick. Women dated less frequently and the median age at marriage was 20. Andrew Cherlin quotes a *New York Times Magazine* expert from 1953: "A girl who hasn't a man in sight by the time she is 20 is not altogether wrong in fearing that she may never get married."[52] The race was on. Thus commentators would urge women to consume to make themselves ideal romantic partners and win the competition for eligible men as soon as possible. The following excerpts are drawn by Bailey from a selection of magazines at the time:

> If you are not gifted with a perfect figure and flawless skin, there is only one solution for you. You must apply yourself relentlessly to the task of making nature over so that you can take your place without self-consciousness in the race for a husband.

> The modern world has given you a billion dollar cosmetic industry, diet experts, specialized stylists and brand-new psychological knowledge; all to storm the barricades of bachelorhood.[53]

Consumption of modern beauty products thus became a cultural requirement for young women wanting to look beautiful enough to attract a husband. In these ways, then, single and married women "were produced as the ideal subjects of consumption in twentieth century America"[54] and around the world. Beliefs about women's love of shopping and ideas such as "women's retail therapy" or "shopping making women feel better"[55] in the United States and elsewhere have now acquired the status of "common sense." In the chapters that follow, I will show the globalized nature of these processes by showing how similar dynamics were at play among young Luo women, seemingly as far removed historically and culturally from twentieth- and twenty-first-century US women as one can imagine.

In the contemporary West, young women's consumption is tied not just to (post)modernity, but to power. Young women in particular continue to be targeted and produced as consumers. Anita Harris argues, for example, how "the reinvention of youth citizenship as consumer power has been largely enacted through young women. Girls have become the emblem of this consumer citizen."[56] She goes on to note, "Young women are also positioned as excellent choice makers, having taken the gains of feminism, such as increased freedoms, assertiveness, and economic independence, and applied them to the market. Their confidence and success are frequently measured by their purchasing power. In the words of one journalist, 'Girl power is flexing its economic muscles' via the spending power of 'single professional, independent and confident young women.'"[57] In this way, she argues, Girl Power is problematically conflated with consumption. Feminist ideals of young women's independence from men are exploited to facilitate young women's active engagement in consumption. As "Girl Power" ideals get exported to developing countries, I will show in chapter 5 how key social institutions such as schools have become crucial enablers of young women's transformation into consuming women and modern (read: consumer) citizens.

## FUNDING WOMEN'S CONSUMPTION

How, however, has and is women's consumption being paid for? To be sure, women's economic independence and thus their ability to fund their own consumption have markedly improved. In the United States, women's labor-force participation rates increased rapidly over the twentieth century. While only 6% of married and 40% of single women worked in 1900, it was not until 1980 that more than 50% of married women participated in the labor force. Women were largely involved in part-time jobs or low-paying jobs in the service industry or in nursing, teaching, and clerical work. By 2000, labor-force participation rates of married and single women were 60% and 70%, respectively, with little change since then.[58] Many married women work in part-time jobs in order to juggle both child-care as well as work, and thus are not the primary breadwinners. The gendered inequality in wages continues, with full-time wage-earning women earning 80% of men's pay.[59] In sum, even while both men and women are drawn into consumer cultures, women were and are generally still unequal to men in their financial ability to consume; yet, critically, they are cultivated to have greater consumer wants, needs, and desires compared to men, for expenditures not just on the household and on their children, but also on themselves.[60] How do women deal with this imbalance? Arguably, for much of the twentieth and early twenty-first century, women's economic dependence on and ability to persuade providing men to fund them was *built into* their cultivation as consuming women.

The consequences of these globalized dynamics for consuming young women in production in Africa are tragic. As the ranks of the middle and upper classes across Africa have grown in the postcolonial era, inequalities have become exacerbated. Extreme wealth is increasing alongside extreme poverty; this means that, as noted in chapter 1, modernity and the consumer goods that signify it openly and regularly beckon, but few can afford them independent of providing men, as I will show in chapter 6. Nyamnjoh, in describing young women's transactional sex relationships in Senegal, Cameroon, and Botswana, went as far as noting, "as everywhere the global tele-evangelism of consumption is converting Africans into various degrees of consumerism and seeking to mold especially youth into consumer zombies."[61]

## CONCLUSION

Gendered disparities in HIV rates are at least in part the result of what happens when modern consumption desires and gendered and generational access to income combine with changes in ways of doing love and marriage. The extensively documented accounts of transactional relationships, coupled with widespread gendered disparities in youth HIV rates, suggest that two key factors lie at the root of young women's HIV rates: the *entanglement of love and money*, and *the production of consuming women*. This book examines the nature of this entanglement and production both at a microlevel, showing how the desire for money and gifts becomes inextricably linked with relationships, and at a macrolevel, highlighting how the engine of transactional relationships—the desire for modern consumption—serves as a key mechanism driving young women into the arms of older men with money and higher rates of HIV. In the next chapter, I will show the historical antecedents of these processes among the Luo, before showing how they unfolded in young women's lives.

# 3 Historical and Cultural Context

Individuals who enjoy good health rightly think of themselves as fortunate: But luck has little to do with the broad
patterns of disease and mortality that prevail in each society. The striking variations in health conditions among
countries and cultural groups reflect differences in social
and physical environments. And increasingly, the forces
that shape health patterns are set in motion by human
activities and decisions. *Indeed in creating its way of life,
each society creates its way of death.*

Peter Eckholm

## *AYAKI MATIEKA:* DEATH AND HIV/AIDS AMONG THE LUO

Toward the end of my fieldwork, on a hot Kisumu day, as I sat in a *matatu*
waiting for it to fill up with passengers before taking me and my assistant
Rose to our next interview, it occurred to me to investigate the etymology
of the Luo word for HIV/AIDS, *ayaki*. For languages to stay current and
useful, new words have to be invented in that language—for example, a
computer or the mouse that accompanies it. AIDS was a "new" disease, so
I wondered where its name had come from and what meaning was attached
to that name. Rose's answer was startling. *Ayaki* came from the root *yako,*
which means to consume very fast, in such a way that displays greed. The
word was meant to describe what HIV/AIDS does; when the disease gets to
you, it finishes you very fast. The Luo were no strangers to premature
death. Infant and child mortality had long been high due to malaria, which
was endemic in this region, along with a variety of infectious childhood
diseases. Indeed, Nyanza province has had the worst mortality rates for

children under five in Kenya for the last decade and a half. Between 1993 and 2009, almost one in five children on average died before their fifth birthday.[1] Luo male migrant deaths from road accidents in their back-and-forth journeys between work and home during the 1980s were so ubiquitous that their grieving wives were called "road widows."[2] There seemed to be no rhyme or reason to someone dying. If it was not a road accident, it was malaria; if not malaria, it was cholera. People were dying all the time, and HIV—with its long incubation period of six to ten years before full-blown symptomatic AIDS—was by no means the most immediate killer. However, by the 2000s, the transition from invisible high HIV-prevalence levels (where many were HIV positive but had no visible signs of their illness) to widespread and constant AIDS-related mortality led people to say, often in despair, *"ayaki matieka,"* meaning AIDS is eating us up, consuming us greedily, or finishing us very fast. Death had become greedy. In this chapter, I examine what has become a common way of death among the Luo. I describe the history of the HIV epidemic, the social experience of death, and specific cultural practices exacerbating its spread, as well as cultural explanations for AIDS. I then examine the historical precedents for these high HIV rates by exploring historical transitions to adulthood as they intertwined with structures, dynamics, and ways of life among the Luo. In particular, I will argue that money and consumption provided the link between Luo ways of life and this way of death.

The disproportionate and early burden of the HIV/AIDS epidemic in sub-Saharan Africa was in the region around Lake Victoria, Africa's largest freshwater lake, and the source of the River Nile. Many of the hardest hit locations in the 1980s and 1990s were in lakeside districts and provinces in Uganda (Rakai district), Tanzania (Mwanza and Bukoba provinces), and Kenya (Nyanza province), where the first cases of HIV/AIDS in this area were reported.[3] Current data suggest that this heavy toll has not altered even after three decades, suggesting that the epidemic is now endemic to the region. Nyanza and the Luo have the highest provincial and ethnic group HIV rates in Kenya. As illustrated in figures 3 and 4 in chapter 1, one in six women (16%) and one in ten men (11.4%) in Nyanza province were HIV positive; among the Luo, one in five Luo women (22.8%) and one in six Luo men (17.1%) were HIV positive. The persistently high HIV rates in this region were reflected in the death rates recorded in Nyanza, where AIDS is the main cause of death, despite the introduction between 2003 and 2008 of antiretroviral drugs which prolong the lives of people living with HIV. The therapy has contributed to a slowdown of deaths; however, in a study conducted in 2008 among those aged 15–49, AIDS accounted for 40% of male deaths, with peak mortality at age 35–49, and 50% of female deaths, with peak mortality among those aged 25–34.[4] Thus, women were dying at higher rates and younger ages from AIDS than men.

The reality of these statistics was reflected in a phrase I encountered early and often in fieldwork: "You are either infected or affected." My most acute experience of the density of death occurred in one of the districts I returned to several times during fieldwork. During one focus group interview, students noted:

KATHY: [When] we were still first years, at least every Friday, coffins, more than five were [passing]. So we got scared. . . . Then you come [to] hear that lecturer So-and-So was in this college, he died, the wife died. Now the children are just here. You find this one [hear about someone else], now he's from a funeral, the husband has died of AIDS.

MARY: Yeah, we got scared.

JULIE: Yeah, in fact this is the only year that no student has died of HIV/AIDS. Because they used to die even during exams.

A few weeks later, on the morning of my return to the main district town, the students' words came to life as I was passed by one funeral procession while walking uphill along the main road to my roadside lodging (similar to a one story motel with a row of self-contained rooms) to deposit my luggage, and another when I was on my way back down to the main town to get transport to go to my next interview. In the first funeral procession, a group of cows was escorted by three or four men, with one man blowing a whistle and another holding a spear and directing the cows down the hill. In this act, symbolic of the deceased having been a man well liked in his village, different villagers would contribute a cow to the procession to the funeral. The second procession was composed of a line of speeding vehicles, with their fronts decorated with grass, each blaring their horns and full of people shouting and making as much noise as possible. The vehicles circled the town center before heading back out again.

These two incidents seemed to throw into relief several other things I had noticed during my time traversing this district: the furniture store by the gas station where coffins were now a prominent feature, and a more lucrative item for local carpenters than sofas; seeing two branches of a store named Classic Coffins, which suggested that business had been successful enough to expand; and the cumulative stories of loss—everyone, it seemed, had lost someone, or was losing someone, or was taking care of children who had lost a parent or supporting a relative who had lost someone. It became common for respondents and key informants in this and other districts to mention a funeral they went to last week, or one they were going to that weekend. Additionally, many of the adults who had died left behind children. By 2004, Nyanza province had 388,064 orphans, 25% of Kenya's orphan population.[5] Many people were housing one or more AIDS orphans; stories of grandmothers taking care of their many grandchildren, having lost all their sons and daughters-in-law to AIDS, cumulated. Children living in the many child-headed homes would leave school at the end of the day, and return home to find "the graves waiting for them."[6] Teachers noted that a quarter to three-quarters of the students in their schools were single orphans (who had lost one parent) or double orphans (who had lost both parents). As I visited one school for an interview, a student was in the principal's office being informed of their parent's death; in the middle of an individual interview at another school, a single orphan informed me that her remaining parent had died the week before. So intertwined was the experience of death and AIDS in everyday life.

## CULTURAL PRACTICES AND WAYS OF UNDERSTANDING AIDS

As fieldwork progressed, it became clear that *ayaki* was not the only way the Luo were making sense of all this death. In some settings, people discussed what was happening by talking about *chira*. The Luo described *chira* as a wasting disease (thus similar to some AIDS symptomatology) that people got when they broke social taboos or were guilty of moral transgressions such as not conforming to particular cultural practices and not showing proper respect to particular individuals such as mothers. For many, it was not that they did not believe that HIV caused AIDS; rather, in a similar fashion to that found by Evans-Pritchard among the Azande,[7] while everyone might understand that someone got HIV through unprotected sex with an HIV-infected person, the *socially relevant* question was why that person, at that time, in that place? HIV, after all, is not indiscriminate. Further, even in high HIV-prevalence societies (such as this one), most people do not get HIV/AIDS. Scholars argue that in some ways the Luo community was using *chira* as a way to incorporate the new and devastating phenomenon of AIDS within existing cultural frameworks of intelligibility. Since AIDS was largely the result of sex, *chira* was in some ways not just about not following and upholding traditional practices and values, but also a social commentary and curse on sex out of place—premarital sex, illicit sex, incestuous sex, sex with the wrong people, and so on. Thus, commenting on Marjorie Macgoye's book *Chira*, Muriungi notes, "Chira helps people in this community to convert the chaos of symptoms of HIV/AIDS into a recognizable, culturally validated condition with a name, a known cause, treatment and prognosis."[8]

Among middle-aged and older women, there was also social pressure to engage in cultural practices that placed many at risk of acquiring HIV. After a husband had died, "sexual cleansing" was sometimes practiced. Here, a widow had to have sex with a man assigned the task of ridding her of her husband's ghost. Another practice was wife inheritance—where a widow was inherited by a male relative of her deceased husband. The original intent of this practice was to create a "corporate safety net" for the widow and her children and keep them within the protection of the family, and enable a widow to stay within the clan lineage and on her husband's land. Additionally, if she did not have children at the time of her husband's death, children resulting from a sexual relationship with the inheritor would become heirs of her husband's land.[9] However, both sexual cleansing and wife inheritance put a widow not already infected with HIV at risk of acquiring it. These practices have become further distorted in recent years by the rise of local commercial industries around widow inheritance and other sex-related rites. Perhaps because of the fear of HIV further spreading within the extended family, families who no longer want to perform these roles themselves have started to hire men (*joter*) to inherit widows and perform sexual cleansing. Thus, while middle-aged and older men and young women have the highest rates of HIV in this and other settings and are the main focus of this study, these persisting cultural practices place middle-aged and older Luo women and these hired young men at risk of HIV acquisition and transmission.[10]

There were also several indications that this was a "sex-positive" culture. Sexually suggestive Luo songs were often played on public transportation vehicles, and in different settings respondents would note that sex was woven into many cultural activities and rites to fulfill customs. As one respondent put it, "[sex] crowns all the activities," meaning that sex was a fitting end to many activities. In an extended conversation with one focus group, for example, several such customs were detailed that were more likely to be practiced in rural areas of Nyanza in particular:

> When people start digging their *shambas* [farms], a lady is needed [for sex], when crops are being harvested, a lady is needed. . . . A new house is built, a lady is needed to crown it. So in the Luo culture there is the issue of building a cottage, the first house. So maybe you were married but you had not actually built this one. So you are being told that once you build this, your wife cannot be the first woman. So you have to look for another woman to spend [the night] with in this [house], [after] that is when your wife can come in. When your parents die, after three days there must be sex.

These types of sex-related customs associated with particular seasons and rituals were corroborated by discussions I had with some key informants throughout my fieldwork.[11] It is important to note, however, the disagreements that existed about what were the "true" customs and traditions. For example, others argued that the real tradition was that sex with anyone *other than* one's wife or wives would bring about *chira* in the opening of a home. Thus, there was a sense that some of these were simply convenient and creative "reinventions" of traditions stated by men to justify extramarital or concurrent sex, which had not been previously sanctioned outside of polygamous marriages based on bride wealth.

## "THEY KNOW BUT THEY IGNORE"?

The landscape was full of HIV-prevention and AIDS-awareness media. Towns and roadways were littered with billboards and painted signs

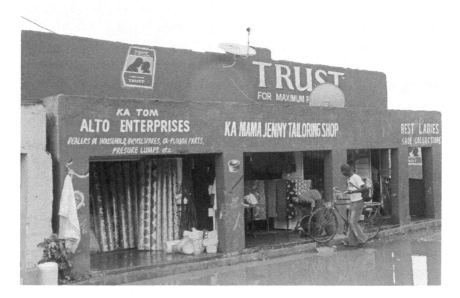

*Figure 9.* Trust Condom sign. Photograph by Jackson Wanga.

encouraging safe sex and HIV testing. Low-cost condoms were widely available and sold in many of the small kiosks where locals bought their groceries and engaged in other shopping. (See figure 9.)

Even youth in some of the most remote schools I visited (some requiring two public transportation vehicles and a walk inland several hours long to get to) asked technical questions about condoms at the end of interviews. Plenty of HIV voluntary counseling and testing (VCT) clinics were located throughout the province, and overall millions of dollars had been spent on a variety of HIV-prevention campaigns in Nyanza.[12] After three decades, there was a weariness about HIV/AIDS. People were tired of talking about it, and NGO workers were frustrated at the lack of progress after years of effort. They had clearly had some success with spreading knowledge and awareness of HIV/AIDS and how to prevent acquiring it, but little of this knowledge seemed to have translated into action, at least as evidenced by the HIV-prevalence rates. Thus, in trying to understand the high HIV rates in Nyanza, widespread ignorance of AIDS and AIDS-related mortality does not seem to be a particularly compelling explanation. Rather, a respondent's noting that "they know but they ignore" seemed to best encapsulate the apparent gap between knowledge and behavior.

Funerals were a classic illustration of this gap. I first briefly describe the impact of funerals on the Luo before discussing how paradoxical they were. Going to funerals had become a frequent weekend activity for many respondents, and many suspected AIDS as the cause of death for the person they were going to bury. (Continued stigma meant that it was not always publicly announced.) The sheer expense of funerals was reflected in respondents' description of the diminished scale of the occasions over the past several years as the numbers of funerals in communities began to escalate.[13] Where before entire cows were slaughtered for funeral guests, now it would be a goat or a sheep, or smaller portions of meat would be bought at a store. Thus, while funerals were lucrative for carpenters and other funeral service providers, the costs of several funerals within one extended family over short periods of time, including constant and expensive travel to and from different parts of the province and country as well as coffins and attendant burial expenses, and the need to support those who were left behind by the deceased meant that they were ultimately impoverishing for families.

What was striking about Luo funerals, for an outsider at least, was the fact that they were treated not just as an occasion for sorrow, but also as an occasion for celebrating life. A funeral reminded everyone that life was not a rehearsal. Rather than funerals being a reminder of mortality and the importance of trying to preserve their own life, they often seemed more a reminder to enjoy life since they could die at any time. The constancy of death seemed to have led to a sense of fatalism and an increased incentive to enjoy their life while they were still alive. For women, funerals were occasions to dress up. Women (or their husbands) would buy new cloth, which they would then take to a tailor to make into extravagant outfits that they could wear at funerals. Youth in particular seemed to behaviorally defy the known reality of AIDS at funerals. At funeral wakes, young men in some communities would fight over who would pursue potentially HIV-infected widows for transactional "sugar mummy" or "marriage-like" relationships.[14] Young men and women described looking forward to all-night funeral dance parties (*nyati adero*) as a prime opportunity to meet same-aged partners and engage in casual hookups,[15] even while they noted that many of those they saw dying of AIDS were young people close in age to them. When asked to be specific not just about age but also about gender, many young people would say that it was young women they saw dying the most. Their actions at funerals, then, belied their knowledge of this statistical (as documented earlier) and empirical reality that they were observing unfold: that women were dying at younger and higher rates than men. Thus, it seems that when people lamented *ayaki matieka,* implicit in the statement was the recognition that AIDS was not consuming just anyone; it was consuming young women.

## HISTORICAL TRANSITIONS TO ADULTHOOD

In order to understand how AIDS became a major way of death among the Luo, and among young women in particular, it is worth first exploring their ways of life, as Eckholm suggests in the epigraph opening the chapter. In this next section, I explore the historical precedents of social-structural processes that shaped transitions to adulthood among the Luo between the 1950s and 1980s. I rely on both historical accounts, as well as the experiences of my middle-aged and older respondents, aged 45–93. I do not attempt here a comprehensive account of the Luo; rather, I focus more specifically on how youth came of age, their relationship-formation processes culminating in marriage, the changing socioeconomy on which it depended, and consequent shifts in attitudes toward mass education, salaried employment, money, and consumption all aimed toward attaining *raha* (the good life) and the ideal Luo way of life.[16] I will illustrate how, in the end, money and consumption were not only seen as a necessary support to the *raha* way of life, but also served as a key pathway to the AIDS way of death.

### Coming of Age and Relationship-Formation Processes

Many of my middle-aged and older respondents grew up in compounds or homesteads comprising their father, his wife (or wives), their unmarried siblings, their married brothers and their wives, and other relatives.[17] Each wife had to have her own house in which she lived with her young children; as a result, one compound would and still typically has several households and many related residents. An important house within the compound was that of Pim—a grandmother or older female relative past childbearing. While most young children, regardless of gender, stayed with their mother, at around five years of age they moved into Pim's household *(siwindhe)*. Pim's role was to educate the children under her care. Young boys stayed with Pim until puberty, at which point they moved out and, together with other boys in the compound, built their own *simba*, a bachelor hut they all shared. While they ate with their own mothers, they spent the night in their *simba*. When an older boy in the *simba* got married, the *simba* would become his house, and younger boys would have to move out and build a new *simba* for themselves.[18] While boys' learning and transition would proceed under the tutelage of male elders and older boys in the community, Pim's role in preparing young girls for marriage and motherhood—key ways in which they were recognized as women—continued once the boys had left. In Pim's household, girls would be taught both practical skills such as household management, as well as social skills such as the management of sexuality and relationships with boys.[19] Girls were encouraged to visit young men in their *simbas*, and sometimes even spend the night, pairing off and engaging in thigh sex (where the young man would insert his penis back and forth between his partner's thighs for stimulation), which Pim had taught the girls how to do.[20] The girls were meant to police one another, ensuring that full penetrative (vaginal) sex did not occur. There were also many village dances, particularly at funerals, which provided many opportunities for youth to socialize and get to know one another.[21] Since these dances were all-night affairs, they provided personal time for couples without oversight or chaperoning. However, many historical accounts note that virginity was prized, and they describe virginity inspections conducted by the groom's older brother and the bride's sister. After the couple consummated the relationship, a fire was lit and the groom's penis inspected for blood. If there was blood, there would be much celebration as they returned to the bride's home, not only because of the bride's virginity, but also because of the extra cattle that could now be included in the bride price. If there was no blood, the return home was marked by silence and a sense of shame.[22] However, it is clear that there were, in fact, many culturally sanctioned opportunities for spending time with young men where virginity could be lost. Indeed, one of the things Pim taught her charges was "methods of contraception—both by magical means and by practical means, and how to procure an abortion if [the girl] was prepared to risk the consequences of breaking the rules. The herb used to procure an abortion is a very powerful purgative which also contracts the womb, but an overdose would be fatal."[23]

A common story I was told by many middle-aged and older women was that Pim told them they would be married to an old man if they got pregnant before marriage.[24] Since a girl could continue to visit different men in their *simbas* until the bride price was fully paid, it might not always be clear who the father was, and a young man could easily disclaim paternity and refuse to marry the girl. Taboos about an unmarried girl giving birth in her natal household meant that she was likely to be married off quickly to an older man as his third or fourth wife.[25] It thus appears that sexuality was governed in a much looser fashion in the past than was often portrayed by older people. Historical accounts show a striking similarity to elders' perceptions of current youth sexuality. The picture these elders paint of the promiscuous youth of today compared to the chaste youth of the past does not appear to be entirely accurate.[26] The fact that virginity was checked at all suggests that it was not a status taken for granted; even then, it was apparently recognized that some girls had premarital sex and some did not. Indeed, it appears that a young woman had to walk a fine line between entertaining a variety of men, as was culturally expected, and avoiding pregnancy—at least until she found her husband.

For both men and women, marriage was a major marker of adulthood. In the DIIS survey, among those born between 1950 and 1974, at least half the women were married by age 17 while at least half the men were married by age 23; this was about a five-year age gap between young men's and women's median age at first marriage. About a third (31%) of women and a quarter (24%) of men in this age group were involved in polygamous marriages.[27] Polygamy was a particularly prized form of marriage among men, though few could afford it. Marrying many wives could only be accomplished through having wealth, since the bride price had to be paid and a house had to be built for each wife. Polygamy was prized because it presented the path to male political power. A man with many wives was also a man with alliances in several kinship and clan groups (since a man could not marry someone in his own kinship or clan group); he thus had a high status, having had experience in dealing with the politics of a large household. He could also serve as a neutral party in conflict—close enough to and trusted by the people concerned (because he had married one of their daughters), but distant enough because he was from a different clan. Having several wives was also economically sensible; more hands were available to farm the land, and when one wife was pregnant, the others could compensate for lost labor.[28]

The first marriage was processual, carried out in a series of stages. The couple was likely to have met at a dance, or when a group of girls had visited a group of men in their *simba*. If a young man liked a girl, he would first ask the girl and, if she consented, would return to her home, this time with friends and relatives, with someone designated to carry out negotiations for the bride price. If these were successfully concluded, a ritual was carried out where there was a mock abduction of the bride: young men from the groom's side went to Pim's house where the girl was and dragged her off. The girl would scream and struggle and make it look like she did not want to go.[29] Once they left the home, she would cease protest. Shortly after, girls from her home would follow.

Consummation of the marriage and checking for virginity (noted earlier) would occur that evening. The bride would stay at the groom's place temporarily, but once he started paying the bride price, she would be encouraged by her family to return home as frequently as possible until he had paid everything in full, at which point she could stay with her husband permanently. A concluding ceremony—*riso*—then occurred and was considered the final act of marriage.[30] The anthropologist Evans-Pritchard described the Luo process of marriage in 1950 this way:

> The husband, or his father begins to pay bride wealth and the wife's parents put pressure on him to expedite payment by encouraging their daughter to return home on frequent visits. The husband cannot prevent her departure, nor can he demand her return. . . . The husband pays an animal, then the wife returns to her parents, then he pays another animal, and so on, till the parents are satisfied and let him take his wife for good. . . . As the husband is anxious to start a home of his own and cannot do so while his wife is constantly running back to her parents he now pays the cattle as fast as he can.[31]

## THE CHANGING SOCIOECONOMY AND THE GROWING
## NEED FOR MONEY

As we can see from the description of the marriage process, having wealth was critical to attaining this crucial marker of adulthood, and certainly to acquiring more than one wife. Bride wealth was reckoned in exchange of animals in this and many other African cultures.[32] Cattle in many African societies at the time were "the supreme form of property . . . they could congeal, store and increase value, holding it stable in a world of flux. [They were] gross, slow moving units of trade."[33] A Luo man with many cattle was considered a man with a lot of wealth, and cattle's importance to the Luo socioeconomy[34] meant that a major form of a young man's labor was herding cattle, essentially taking care of the wealth that would eventually secure him his bride. Among women, farming was a key form of labor; this was mainly for subsistence and not a major source of wealth. Many elders I interviewed said, "the Luo are not farmers." Ocholla-Ayayo, a noted Luo scholar, remarked, "although they cultivate the land in order to produce an adequate food supply, this is done from necessity in most cases and not out of devotion."[35]

Another aspect of the Luo socioeconomy was fishing, though this was not a significant source of income earlier in the twentieth century. Fishermen were considered of a lower status than men who owned cattle. The Luo called themselves *jonam* (people of the lake), and they also engaged in several lake-based entertainment activities such as competitive rowing. However, while they were drawn to the lake for these reasons, population density was higher in "fertile northerly locations" than it was by the lake in the early twentieth century.[36] These locations were likely more ideal for cattle grazing. By the 1980s, three decades later, however, a reversal had occurred and population density in Nyanza was much higher near the lake.[37] This reflected increased agriculture, which was helped by proximity to the lake, as well as the rapid growth of the fishing industry. Many historians attribute this increasing shift to fishing and agriculture to rinderpest epidemics between the 1880s and 1920s, which decimated the cattle population and made it difficult for people to replenish their stocks.[38] This was a major shock to the Luo socioeconomic system, more so because it was followed by the introduction by the British colonialists of the hut tax (property tax), payable only in coin and cash.[39]

Given the domestic set up of Luo homes, and the multiple huts within the compound of the family patriarch, this effectively created a large demand for money to meet tax obligations. For Luo families, and men in particular, there was a new dilemma: cash-crop production or labor migration out of the province. Attempts by the colonial and postcolonial governments to encourage the Luo to engage in cash-crop production, however, were not very successful, particularly in areas with higher population density and thus smaller lots. Smaller lots prevented the possibility of large-scale production that would result in bigger returns. For many Luo, labor migration was a more attractive solution; they realized that they could get a better income if they worked for someone else outside the province than if they tried to grow cash crops. This resulted in between a quarter and a half of the young men migrating out for work by the mid-twentieth century, leading one commentator to note, "Central Nyanza has therefore developed into a major exporter of labor."[40] This had long-term consequences that persist today, in the absence of fathers, brothers, and other male relatives, as well as in the predominance of women in subsistence agricultural farming at home and their need to gain their own financial footing when remittances are not regular and when the crop is failing.[41] Cultivating an adequate food supply was made more difficult when maize was introduced as a replacement for sorghum, a hearty grain. As the historians Cohen and Atieno Odhiambo document, while sorghum was more resistant to periods of infrequent and inadequate rainfall, maize was less so; thus crop failure occurred more frequently.[42] *Nikech kech* (because of hunger)—a recurring motif in my community interviews when I asked about general issues in the community as an icebreaker—was a common motivation given for the otherwise undesirable actions of others. As a result, there was increased dependence on other sources for income to buy food and alleviate hunger. There were varied agricultural innovations among women early in the twentieth century as they tried to build up agricultural surpluses, which could then be converted to other forms of wealth. However, as soil fertility declined and yields alongside them, women increasingly turned to other forms of labor such as buying and selling bananas and fish for income generation.[43]

## CULTURAL CONSEQUENCES OF LABOR MIGRATION

Several cultural consequences resulted from men's large-scale labor migration out of Nyanza. Many Luo men were living among people of different ethnic groups and cultures while working for white colonialists on farms, in railway construction, in the civil service, and so on. As a result, these male migrants—*jopango*—were "crucial communicators of culture."[44] On their return home for visits, they would bring back with them new innovations, new ideas, new styles, and the goods that went along with them, in addition to the income that could purchase these things. New standards were set by the *mzungu* (the white man). "In terms of superlative reference, the mzungu became the man of culture par excellence, the one to whom all deferred, the subject of so much conversation at the places of employment . . . you dressed well like a mzungu, or you spoke English well like a mzungu, or even if you spoke Dholuo [the Luo ethnic group language] particularly distinctively, you were said to speak like a mzungu."[45] This fed into demands for the increased consumption of products requiring cash income (such as clothing) in addition to a shift in diet toward eating meat (which they had to buy) away from vegetables (which they grew themselves) and fish (which were bartered with fishermen).[46]

These new standards also spilled over into changing ideals about what constituted a beautiful woman. Writing in the late 1950s, Shadrack Malo, a respected Luo elder, in his classic book on Luo customs and practices profiled the ideal Luo woman, who reflected the colonial influence on men's tastes and concepts of beauty, yet who was a curious mixture of the traditional and the modern:

> Today's Luo man looks for different things in a woman. He looks at the physical features, her academic achievements and her economic ability. He looks for the following:
>
> a)  Is she brown or light skinned?
> b)  Does she look good in powder, *onego poda* (all made up and dressed up) (sic)
> c)  Is her neck long?
> d)  Is she slender and looks good in clothes

e) Is her teeth white (sic)

f) Does she have a gap, *singare*

g) Is she educated

h) Does she speak good English

i) Is she a teacher, a leader of women's group

j) Did she pass Cambridge O level certificate [reaching form 4]

k) Has she been abroad to America, London or Europe[47]

In some respects, these sets of ideals reinforced older conceptions of beauty—a long neck, white teeth, and a gap between the two front teeth. The last ideal in particular, going abroad, resonated with a man's desire to marry into a wealthy family and thus bring the seeds of wealth into his own family through the children that would be born.[48] In other respects, these ideals made radical breaks from older conceptions of beauty among the Luo—from dark skin to brown or light skin and to the use of powder and makeup. Migrants discussed beauty "in terms of *kwar ka nyar Goa* (being brown like a Goan girl) or *ber ka nya Silisili* (being as beautiful as a Seychellois)."[49] Education, good English, and being a professional were now considered ideals. This Western standard of style and being, along with the consumption required to meet this standard, has remained, as we shall see in subsequent chapters; and there was a sense in which the socioeconomy had been *reorganized* to these new ends.

These shifting ideals and the lifestyle they gave birth to seemed to be encapsulated in a phrase I came across over and over from both Luo and non-Luo throughout my fieldwork—*gihero raha* (they love pleasure). This reflected the Luo love for "the good life." To this end, the Luo were "not afraid of spending" to achieve the good life or pleasure. Wealth accumulation was not so important since life was seen as too short. As one teacher told me, "the life of wealth creation is boring for us." It was more important to have fun and enjoy life. Someone from the Kikuyu ethnic group, he went on to say, could be renting out good houses but living in a shack; but this was "not for a Luo." Life was to be enjoyed. There are many Luo sayings about enjoying life. A common one was *dhiang tho gilum edhoghe* (a cow dies with grass in the mouth), and another was *kwer tuo mane puotho* (the hoe dies while digging). Both of these sayings suggested that people

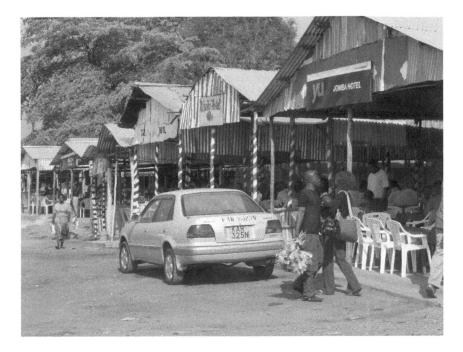

*Figure 10.* Hotels by the lake. Photograph by Jackson Wanga.

would continue doing what they enjoyed until the day they died. In one interview, a non-Luo girl noted, "we believe that most Luo men are somehow lifists | that is, life-ists] . . . they are somehow extravagant." These sayings are not far from the familiar saying "eat, drink and be merry, for tomorrow we die." Enjoying and living life to the fullest and to the best of one's financial ability encapsulated the best way to live. A key vehicle for attaining *raha* was consumption. Thus, in contemporary times, people living closest to the lake were seen as best embodying *raha;* rich from daily sales of fish, and confident of getting more money the next day, they could spend their money at the many hotels, bars, and tailoring shops that lined the streets of lakeside towns. (See figure 10.)

As a side note, it is worth noting that such cultural ideals, while seemingly trivial, can be real in their consequence and in motivating individuals or groups to strive for these valued ends, regardless of whether those ends are actually achievable by the majority of people, and regardless of what they might actually cost. A classic example is the so-called American dream,[50] itself an ideal that is consumptive at heart: the idea that if you work hard, you will have the income to consume products that exemplify your achievement—for example, owning a home complete with a white picket fence, an SUV or two in the driveway, a big screen TV in the basement man cave to watch the big game, and money to take the kids to Disneyland.

The persistence of these stereotypes of the Luo as a people who love and live for *raha,* both in how they are portrayed by others, and in how they portray themselves, is striking. The culture of consumption, of *kula raha* (eating or consuming pleasure), Atieno Odhiambo notes, was fueled by the growth of an African middle class earning decent wages for the first time in Nairobi, Kenya's capital in the mid- to late 1950s.[51] While this culture surely enveloped urbanites of all ethnicities, Luo migrants in the city were seen as having most fully appropriated the *raha* lifestyle, defined as "the enjoyment of alcohol, music, food, good clothes and sex—even during the bad times."[52] That it was a stereotype and was not necessarily reflective of the reality of many Luo was noted in the autobiography of Oginga Odinga, a prominent Luo elder and Kenya's first vice president, which was published in 1967: "I was haunted by the view which other Africans had of the Luo people. I had been hurt at Makerere [a prominent Ugandan and East African university] by the accusations of fellow students from other tribes that the Luo were extravagant, self-centered, and exhibitionist; that they used their money for show and not to improve themselves."[53]

Mboya discusses how tribalism, co-opted for political purposes in post-colonial Kenya, encouraged stereotyping in order to undermine the political ambitions of Luo aspirants. However, he also underscores the complexity of the appropriation of these stereotypes by the Luo and the fact they could become a self-fulfilling prophecy. Focusing on a prominent Luo benga musician of the 1990s, the late Okatch Biggy, he talks about the Luo as "the serious people of *raha,*" as expressed in Biggy's music. Biggy, he argues, fully embraced and sang about the *raha* lifestyle as applied to the Luo. However, he introduced some nuance into the cultural stereotype. Yes, he sang, the Luo thoroughly enjoyed the *raha* lifestyle, but only after engaging in hard work to earn the money to fund it, a primary means of which was excelling in education. Further, earned money, he sang, was also used toward culturally valued ends, such as taking care of the poor and orphans, and sharing wealth with others in the community. The songs were not only an embrace of the stereotype, to the extent that the Luo were going to be stereotyped, but also a reinfusion of the stereotype with "positive tribalism."[54] Thus, if money was honorably earned, and partly used to help the community, what was wrong with spending money to enjoy life?[55]

## THE INCREASING IMPORTANCE OF EDUCATION AND SALARIED EMPLOYMENT

As cash to purchase this lifestyle was increasingly desired (instead of cattle wealth), education began to be seen as an important route to gaining the means to afford a beautiful wife or wives, and to have the money and status to live the good life. This was coupled with what some older male respondents described as the Luo's "employment mentality," which reflects a preference for being formally employed and earning a salary rather than starting and running a business. It is in this light that Nyanza's particular thirst for education and stable employment should be seen.

Initially, school was hated, perceived as a "taint," and treated with suspicion, not least because it created a clash between the "cultured Luo" and the Westernized, schooled Luo.[56] Indeed, school was an institution to which you went by force. As James, an older Luo gentleman in his 80s, recounted to me, "Chiefs were forced to take their children to school and it was like a requirement but they didn't take their [own] children. Instead they looked for people whom they hated most in the community and [sent] their children. They didn't know they were helping these children. They felt they were making them suffer."

Over time, however, the changing socioeconomic conditions described earlier made school begin to look like an attractive pathway to social mobility, jobs, and money, first in the colonial and then the postcolonial era.[57] Thus, even though the tensions noted earlier between the educated and the noneducated persisted, school, which was a fee-paying institution, became increasingly valued.

Among young women, initially, school was not considered a priority, and many stayed home while their brothers went to school. Those who did go to school only got a little education before having to leave to let their siblings have a chance to go to school as well. Janita, a 65-year-old lady who only reached standard 5 (fifth grade),[58] recounted, "after my father died, they said they would only be educating the sons, saying that giving girls small education was better because actually they were just going to get married."

However, among those two decades younger, many young women were able to go slightly further in school. For example, Mary, a middle-aged lady, described reaching as far as Form 4 (tenth grade) before leaving school so that there was money for her siblings to go to school. Lili, who was in her late 40s, was able to reach Form 2 before dropping out because of a lack of money for school fees. Four of her nine siblings were able to complete high school. She noted that it was her mother, who earned a living selling fish, who paid for her school fees, since her father did not support girls' education.

More Luo women born between 1955 and 1974 began primary school (85%) compared to other Kenyan women (77%); however, there was greater attrition throughout the school careers of Luo women. As a result, Luo women had lower rates of entry into high school compared to other Kenyan women.[59] Thus, the Luo were particularly eager for girls' education, compared to other ethnic groups in the country, and this partially reflected shifts in fathers' attitudes toward their daughters' education as the century progressed. However, this shift only occurred to a point; girls' education was halted not only when the cost of their education infringed on that of their brothers, but also when the family thought it was time for them to marry and start their own family.[60] School and marriage were seen as incompatible, and adulthood, defined by marriage and motherhood, could only be postponed for a while. Many older women saw marriage as the reason for their halted education; some were pulled directly from school to their forced marriage, and some married shortly after the end of their schooling.

The increase in young women's schooling, however, also meant the dearth and decline of Pim. Primary schools were often located many miles away from the student's home. This meant that a student's day could be almost entirely taken up by school, including hours walking to the school, hours at school, and then hours returning from school. If a girl went to high school, this was often a boarding school requiring her to be away from home for months at a time. When school was over, as already noted, marriage followed shortly after. This resulted in limited time for Pim to give her charges household and sexual education. While young women sometimes referenced their grandmothers as their source when talking about various cultural customs and taboos, it was rare to hear of Pim described in her traditional role as a more full-time educator during the interview.[61] Indeed, modern mass education in this and other settings, rather than complementing local and ethnic organizations and institutions responsible for teaching youth that began in the precolonial era, seems to be largely replacing them.[62]

More Luo men went to school compared to Luo women. They also began school at higher rates compared to other Kenyan men. Among men born between 1952 and 1974, 13% of non-Luo men reported having no education, compared to 4% of Luo men. However, more Luo men's education ended with primary school graduation, and many of those who began secondary school dropped out. Non-Luo men, however, were more likely to have completed secondary school and gone on to higher education.[63] A major reason for men's attrition from school was lack of money to pay school fees, a situation similar to that of women. As Oduor, an older gentleman, explained, "education was cheap but getting the money was difficult. That's why people like I could not go to school." However, another major reason was that there were jobs available for men even with a few years of education. Another older gentleman, Okwaro, noted that even without passing the exam marking successful completion of primary school, there were jobs available: "When you sat for this exam, even if you failed, you [could] get jobs with the railway, post office, in banks, or [from] the Asian [businessmen]. . . . The work that a [primary] Class 5 [student] could do then, . . . a Form 4 [high school graduate] of today could not do. A Form 1 and 2 were considered [very] educated. Tom Mboya [a famous Luo politician], for example, reached Form 2." In this description, Okwaro shows the low educational bar for formal sector jobs in the early postcolonial era, compared to contemporary educational requirements for similar positions. The demand for people to fill the posts left behind by colonialists as Kenya transitioned into independence in 1963 was high.[64] A young man did not have to go far in his schooling to see the material returns of his education in terms of salaried jobs and income.

## CONTRADICTIONS OF MONEY AND CONSUMPTION

The gradual shift in the medium of exchange from cattle to cash was not seen as wholly favorable and was blamed by many of my oldest Luo respondents (age 60–93) for tearing apart the fabric of their community. As Awori, a lady in her 80s, put it, "it is money which has spoilt things"; Mary, in another setting, noted, "money destroys the land." What they were referring to was their perceived undermining of an otherwise deeply engrained Luo value of communalism. In his autobiography, Odinga described how the head of his village solved the problem of food disparities between households during a famine: "He would fetch me late every night and take me from granary to granary to examine the food stocks. When we found a granary with little left in it he would direct me to a granary which had plenty, and we would replenish the almost exhausted store."[65] In describing an event seared in his memory decades after its occurrence, Odinga was illustrating a key value often emphasized among the Luo: that the rich were required to be generous and to share their wealth. If they did not do so, local actions were taken to ensure that they did. These actions reflected communally imposed and regulated obligations between the wealthy and the poor, and served as a safety net and as insurance for the community in times of need. Ong'ombe, an older man, lamented that while in the past when a woman gave birth, fishermen used to give her free fish, now this could never happen. This mutual dependence was also reflected in the barter system that was in place at the time. As Apinyi, an older lady, described, "if I wanted milk and I had millet, I just went to the person with milk and exchanged my millet and then I got the milk . . . with barter, you were only restricted to what the other had." Thus barter trade not only created an interdependence among people in the community—including a willingness to share and exchange what they had—but also limited individual consumption to items that people in one's own community had, or could make, given that one had what they wanted.[66] The shift toward a cash economy, however, radically changed this interdependence. As one elder noted, "now money is what is used as an exchange value so without it you cannot do anything." Another noted, "with the coming of money, you were able to get other things [even if you did not] have millet for milk . . . with money you can have milk."

Money clearly gave people the independence and freedom to break out of local options for products and acquire items that other people in their community did not have. However, money also essentially *created* poverty among those who did not have access to cash. Cash created two groups of people: those who could opt out of the barter economy and those who could not. It created a class of people who could purchase and consume modern products that others in their community with no money could not access, and gave this class an independence and freedom from localized systems of exchange. In the minds of my oldest respondents, who had observed several decades of change, it had dramatic effects on the morality of the community in the process. For example, Obongo said, "[In the past] there was communal love. People loved each other in the community and so somebody could just give another person something free of charge and not demand payment, unlike now. Now there is nothing for nothing. There must be payment in form of money."

As money became the new currency, people could no longer offer what they had to get something they wanted; now they had to use money. While an economy and exchange of animals and things have certainly continued through the present as part of an ancestral, intergenerational, and communal system of entrustment richly described by the anthropologist Parker Shipton,[67] exchanges increasingly began to be characterized by cash. Further, as money became more prized, there arose a division between wealth measured by things that could be shared and wealth measured by things that could not be shared. In his monograph on money among the Luo, Shipton noted, "People with money can live by different rules than people without. Luo who will lend neighbors farm tools or lanterns freely may refuse to lend cash: it is harder to collect. Nothing is more sought after than cash, but nothing disappears more quickly. Cash has created its own morality."[68] He went on to note the features of cash that lent it to this different kind of morality among the Luo: "Several features of cash make it especially risky. One is its concealability . . . another feature is divisibility . . . finally, the transportability and almost universal substitutability of cash make it easier to spend than other, older forms of wealth. All these features combine to produce what we may call a 'private pocket syndrome,' in which family members lose collective control over family wealth."[69]

Thus, in the age of cash that could be stashed in banks and cooperatives, it was not possible to go from granary to granary to check how much people had and then redistribute it. Neither could one see how much wealth a family or person had by the number of cattle and other animals in their backyard. Cash wealth could now be hidden; even within families, collective wealth had become individual wealth. Thus Okoth, an older gentleman, when asked to consider the effect money has had on youth, was able to assign blame to money for its effects on different family relationships:

> Money made girls to become prostitutes, [it is] what has brought AIDS, it is what has spoilt the girls. In this our community, there was no girl who could call a boy, you come. It is there now. It has brought conflict in families. Men like myself cannot let their wives know when they have money, only the saved people like myself can let their wives know that they have money. It has also affected the boys, even becoming thieves. The boy was educated and he didn't get employment . . . so he goes and steals. They are getting into it because they want money for alcohol, to give to girls, for cigarettes, for *bhang* [marijuana]. That's why we say that money has caused problems.

We can see in this statement an elaboration of the kind of change in morality that Okoth thought money introduced. It had affected young women's sexual morality and the communal morality of young men, who no longer respected other people's property. Money also challenged the trust within marriage and brought conflict within families. In his statement, we can also see Okoth setting himself apart from the deteriorating morality by asserting his Christianity when he says, "only the saved people." While in his mind and in the work of other ethnographic observers in the area,[70] there was a clear distinction between the saved and the not saved, the role of Christianity as I encountered it was much more complicated. There was a more syncretic "buffet style" of religion, with a creative mix of traditional African and Christian beliefs and practices that varied among respondents: for example, ancestor worship, keen adherence to rituals to appease spirits, belief in diseases befalling those who did not follow cultural traditions *(chira)*, *in combination with* churchgoing and involvement in local church activities. In other words, Christianity seemed to be part of the larger contemporary Luo cultural toolkit or repertoire, with different pieces of it variously deployed as the occasion warranted.[71] Thus, *both* proponents and opponents of wife inheritance, a traditional cultural practice, could claim Christian support for their position: proponents could point to positive biblical examples of wife inheritance (for example, the story of Ruth), and widows not wanting to be inherited benefited from local church support in building their houses in the face of local opposition to their refusal to conform to traditional customs (support found in the biblical injunction to help widows and orphans).

For many anthropologists, the so-called great transformation effected by money is a common feature of many accounts of the introduction of money into colonial societies.[72] While Georg Simmel, a pioneering sociologist of money, argued that "money acts as an incredibly powerful agent of profound social and cultural transformations,"[73] others dispute the "intrinsic power" attributed to money to enact this transformation. It was not money that alienated or "ushered in moral confusion" or that created alienated social exchange.[74] Rather, they argue that "it is important to understand the cultural matrix into which it is incorporated."[75] As I found in my own interviews excerpted earlier, and as noted by anthropologists of money, "it always seems to be the elders who are deploring the situation."[76] Luo elders' attitudes toward money may merely be an index for their anxieties about other changes to their society, such as declines in durable cattle wealth and the resultant status shifts as pathways to wealth changed. Definitions of who was wealthy began to shift toward those who had the most access to cash money, as opposed to those who had traditional forms of wealth such as owning cattle.

Often, these shifts redistributed power in both generational and gendered ways. New pathways to wealth such as education were pathways that women could also access, and with access to salaried jobs, young men could gain greater access to cash income than their fathers. In both local as well as national perceptions, ownership of radios and TVs and access to running water were increasingly privileged as evidence of wealth over traditional measures. Those wealthy according to "modern" standards would count as wealthy, and those better able to convert their wealth into cash would benefit most from a modernizing economy.[77] Thus, the fisherman would be doing well and experience an upward shift in occupational prestige over the late twentieth century compared to the cattle owner because of the fisherman's greater ability (and need, given how quickly fish rot in the absence of refrigeration, which many did not have) both to convert his "animals" into cash and to quickly replace them by returning to the lake to fish the next day. The anthropologists Maurice Bloch and Jonathan Parry note, across the case studies in their edited volume, "a strikingly similar concern with the relationships between a cycle of short-term exchange which is the legitimate domain of individual—often acquisitive—activity and a cycle of long-term exchanges concerned with the reproduction of the social and cosmic order."[78]

Consequently, in the quotation above from Okoth, we see that his anxieties about money also indexed the dubious short-term ends to which it was now being put by young men (who used their ill-gotten gains "for alcohol, to give to girls, for cigarettes, for *bhang* [marijuana]," as opposed to long-term ends such as bride-wealth payments to their wife's family elders) and young women (who acquired money through transactional relationships and used it on mobile phones, perfumes, and creams, which had become highly desired items for themselves). It seems that how elders described young people's money was as if it were in essence a new example of what Shipton has described as *pesa makech*, or "bitter money." This label was applied to money that was ill gotten, unfair, unjust, or stolen, which was "dangerous to its holder and the holder's family" and was cursed. Nothing good would come to someone in possession of it.[79] This makes sense of Okoth's words that "money made girls to become prostitutes, [it is] what has brought AIDS, it is what has spoilt the girls."

## CONCLUSION

In sum, the pursuit and acquisition of money to fund the good life were seen as mixed blessings. Even though it brought things that were highly valued, it also brought in its wake cultural changes that were destructive. In particular, the problem of HIV among youth, and young women especially, was inextricably linked with the problem of money, as elders saw it. Bitter money and its associated consumption provided the link between the Luo way of life and the Luo way of death. Thus, in reflecting on the meaning of *ayaki matieka* and young women's transactional relationships, it became apparent that young women's consumptive pursuit of *raha* was somehow contributing to the tragic and devastating role HIV played in their early death, certainly in the minds of my respondents. Yet some key questions remained: If so, how and why did consumption become so central to girls on the cusp of adulthood? Why were the HIV/AIDS-prevention strategies of abstinence, being faithful to one partner, and condom use (ABC) that had (apparently) thoroughly saturated the Luo landscape so ineffective in changing young women's HIV risk? Understanding young women's disproportionate HIV risk suggests at the outset a complex interplay between contemporary transitions to adulthood, consumption, and the Luo way of life; subsequent chapters will attempt to unpack this. In particular, above and beyond young women's decisions, I explore how social-structural processes involved in their pursuit of love (chapter 4), education (chapter 5), and a job (chapter 6) both limited and complicated young women's ability to escape their dangerous transition to adulthood.

# 4  Love, Money, and HIV Prevention

Searching for a husband may be as dangerous as finding one.

Shelley Clark

When people embark on intimate relationships, sexually transmitted infections (STIs) are often the last thing on their minds. Further, even as young people select their partners, they are rarely aware of the bird's-eye view or the STI/HIV risk *environment* in which they are making their choices. Yet it is precisely these environments that may turn innocuous, culturally intelligible relationship choices into dangerous ones. As this chapter will illustrate, in Nyanza, the disease environment in which relationship logics governing sexual relationship choices—and nonchoices— unfolded resulted in high risk for young women and protection and temporary safety for young men. I examine how Luo youth characterized their relationships and their motivations underlying their selection of partners. I then show how these characterizations and motivations for young women combined to make the selection of "safe" partners relatively less attractive, at least in the short term, than the selection of "dangerous" partners. I illustrate how the opposite held true for young men. In particular, I show the centrality of money and consumption to the logic of intimate partnership choices and ways of demonstrating love, and I illustrate  how prevention strategies faltered in light of these relationship logics.

## THE HIV RISK ENVIRONMENT

A recent nationally representative study of young US adults found that by age 29, about 16% of men and 37% of women reported having ever had an STI.[1] This STI risk environment in the United States among young people suggests substantial levels of unprotected sex even in a setting where information is widespread, condoms are widely available, income levels are relatively high, and health care is more accessible. Additionally, the statistics reflect the elongated period between first sex and first marriage, where many young adults engage in casual sexual relationships (such as hooking up). In college settings, these relationships are usually alcohol-driven, and condom use may be dispensed if the birth control pill is assumed, and information exchanges—concerning sexual history (or phone numbers)—occur the next day.[2] The big difference between the STI-prevalence findings in the United States and the findings among young people in Luo-Nyanza in figure 11 is that the more prevalent STIs circulating among youth in the United States are mostly curable and rarely fatal.

Figure 11 illustrates trends in HIV-prevalence rates for Luo young women and men in Nyanza. The arrows suggest the risk scenario an HIV-negative teenage girl would be facing in partner selection (which is invisible to her). As shown in the figure, an HIV-negative teenage girl would be at very low risk of encountering an HIV-positive partner if she chose a young man the same age as herself. Gender differences among teenagers are statistically significant.[3] However, any partnership with an older man carries much higher levels of risk. In this risk environment, almost one in ten men aged 20–24 years old, and a third of men aged between 25 and 34 whom a teenage girl might chose would be HIV positive. Thus, a relationship with a sugar daddy—a man 10 years older—would be tragically dangerous. That young Luo women's HIV-prevalence rates closely mirror those of men in their late 20s and early 30s is reflected by the lack of significant gender differences in HIV rates once they transition out of their teens, and it also suggests the age structure of their sexual relationships.[4] In sum, the data illustrate that to get HIV in this setting, teenage girls are most likely having relationships with older partners. It is worth noting two things. First, as noted in chapter 3, and as is also true among contemporary couples in this setting, there is a median five-year gap in young

| Age Group | % HIV Positive | |
| | Women | Men |
| 15–19 | 15.7 | 2.7 |
| 20–24 | 17.4 | 8.5 |
| 25–29 | 34.2 | 28.7 |
| 30–34 | 31.3 | 29.4 |
| TOTAL | 22.3 | 12.5 |

*Figure 11.* HIV prevalence of young Luo-Nyanza women and men, by age group. Source: KDHS 2010.

men's and women's age at first marriage. Thus, partnering with slightly older partners has been and is the norm. Second, it is worth emphasizing that this is a bird's-eye view of the HIV risk environment in Luo-Nyanza. Therefore, while it is immediately evident to us from the figure that some sexual partners were more dangerous than others, it was not necessarily as clear to the young people navigating their romantic lives, nor were they making their choices based on the HIV-prevalence levels of potential partners.[5]

Marriage is a major mechanism for the acquisition and transmission of HIV, and early marriage, under age 20, is a particularly important risk factor.[6] In the DHS survey data from 2010, married teen girls had almost *six times* the HIV rates of unmarried teen girls; further, half of Luo women under 30 had married by age 17. Indeed, in Luo-Nyanza, marriage under the age of 20 among women was the norm. By age 24, virtually all (93%) were married. However, married women in their 20s had HIV rates similar to those of same-aged men.[7] Thus, a major reason for the lack of significant gender differences between the HIV rates of women and men in their 20s and 30s in figure 11 is marriage. While an unmarried girl may easily move from a high-risk to a low-risk partner in the course of her relationship history, a young woman, once married, is locked in to a relationship characterized by frequent and unprotected sex, especially since young women are in their early years of family building.[8]

Thus, for many teenage girls, early marriage played a major role in their HIV acquisition. For unmarried teen girls, while their risk could come from relationships with high-risk teen boys (those with multiple concurrent relationships), they were more likely to encounter HIV in relationships with unmarried or married men in their 20s and older. The data, then, suggest that both premarital *and* marital sexual relationships were risky for young women transitioning to adulthood; the pursuit of love—from the beginning of dating and the sexual debut to finding a husband—was a dangerous proposition.

## ENTANGLEMENTS OF SEX, LOVE, MONEY, AND HIV PREVENTION

### Relationships for Education, Relationships for Sex

As high school–going Luo youth saw it, there were two kinds of romantic relationships: "relationships for education" and "relationships for sex." This distinction first emerged in an interview among a group of schoolboys when I asked whether they had girlfriends. One responded, "I want to ask you something. You are talking about a girl-to-boy relationship? Which kind of relation? Which is concerned to education or concerned to sex?" When I responded that I was interested in both types, they then went on to characterize the two types of relationships. In most cases, both types of relationships were initiated by young men. A relationship for education was usually how relationships began. A couple would "just sit together, or bring our problems or ideas together, then we try to pass them to each other so that we can solve them. Where we are weak the partner may assist." A relationship for sex was different, as Mary noted: "you know there is a boyfriend and a lover, a friend is someone that you can go and visit and you say things that are positive and a lover is that person, let's say that I have gone to see him, what will be in his mind is he will just tell me sweet words, and these sweet words, the main purpose of that man will be just to have sex with me."

Relationships for education were relationships between schoolmates either in the same school or in different schools that were entirely abstinent and almost platonic in nature. It became clear, however, that relationships for education were really the prelude to relationships for sex, and often represented two ends of a continuum with a steady progression from one end to the other. As a high schooler, Tom, noted in explaining why girls may not necessarily put up an argument, "when it is a process, you can't realize. Maybe, at first, you think that it is meant for education . . . but one day you'll just be approached [to have sex] and so their [girls'] saying no will be very difficult because you had been together sharing ideas." With the prior basis of a strong friendship, rejecting sexual advances became difficult for young women. Anything less than "a strong no" could lead to losing their resolve and giving in. Girls said of themselves that their problem was they could be "easily swayed."

Whether or not sex was involved also affected the *duration* of the relationship with a peer, since youth thought relationships involving sex were more likely to involve conflict and be short term in nature. "A friendship of knowledge . . . will go awhile because you'll not have quarrels," a schoolgirl, Akinyi, noted. When I inquired what kinds of quarrels were then characterized by a friendship involving sex, Jane said, "if he fails to satisfy your needs. Maybe you wanted even, let's say, 200 shillings [$2.85] to satisfy your needs. Then here comes a case where he may even tell you that I don't have that [right] now. And then maybe you know that he has the money. Then he is just refusing to give it to you. Then that might end up with quarrels."

While friendships for knowledge or education could last a long time, once sex was introduced, quarrels began. Sex entitled a girl to make claims for gifts or money from a boy, thus changing the relationship in a substantive way. The main subject of quarrels in relationships for sex was over a boyfriend's provision of money and gifts or the lack thereof. Boyfriends with no money or ability to get it could rarely sustain relationships for sex for any length of time. This was the situation in which many young men in school or freshly out of school found themselves. This is important epidemiologically since, because of the fairly low likelihood of getting HIV in a single coital act,[9] the *duration* of a sexual relationship plays a big role in determining disease acquisition. Thus, a young man in a short-term relationship with an HIV-positive partner is at much lower risk compared to one in a long-term relationship, who is regularly exposed to the HIV virus. This might explain why, even though there seemed to be plenty of evidence that teenage men were engaging in sex with young women their age, their HIV rates were very low (2.7%) compared to young women (15.7%). In other words, young men's financial lack and the subsequent short-term relationships were inadvertently protecting them from HIV acquisition.

*Money, Love, and Relationships for Sex*

As seen earlier, in the relationship for education, a couple was "helping" each other and sharing ideas. But once sex entered the picture, the nature of a boy's "help" changed and began to involve helping to raise money for his girlfriend and working different jobs to put the money together for her.[10] However, once she had been helped, her equivalent "help" in return for his labor on her behalf was her having sex with him. Relationships for sex, in other words, were "transactional relationships," where sexual relationships were accompanied by money and gifts. Depending on who one talked to, which came first—the sex or the help—varied; in other words, whether the boy was helping in order to have sex or whether the couple had sex, which then prompted help, varied from youth to youth. Sometimes the way the relationship was described and characterized seemed more like a commercial or quid pro quo exchange. Sidney, for example, felt that most relationships in his school were relationships for sex: "because if a girl comes to a boy for help, for a boy to help her with some amount, that boy will try as much as he can to raise that amount for her, then that boy will also want to enjoy his money. And that is the only way it can happen."

In a similar fashion, Christine said, "sometimes your parents cannot afford some money to buy for us things girls need. So you can go and have sex with a boy so he can give you money to buy your things." For many young men, the only fair exchange or reward for the gift of money was having sex in return. Boys did not necessarily have to be wealthy, but needed to have the ability to get or earn money to help their girlfriends. Before quickly classifying these exchanges as commercial, it is worth delving deeper into the meaning of money in relationships.

It was only in rare cases that youth described relationships for sex which did not involve any gifting of money and were characterized by "pure" love in the ideal-typical Western sense. As Macy said, "You know you can love someone even if he doesn't have money, and then there are those who love a man because they can see he has money, she says, let me eat this one,[11] when the money finishes I will go to another man. So it depends. You can find a man who really doesn't have any money and even when you look at him you see that this one doesn't have money but you still love him." It is interesting that in both cases, a girl "loved" a man, but the reason why she loved him differed. The cultural assumption of the *materiality* of relationships for sex underlies this conception of love.[12] This assumption was also gendered—men were assumed to be the material providers, not women. Love was not just a matter of words; love had to be *demonstrated* and, in this case, demonstrated through the medium of money. For some women, they loved their man because he was able to give them money, and others loved their man for reasons other than his ability to provide. Regardless of the basis for the love, however, most youth and some elders felt that expecting money from a poor boyfriend or from a boyfriend who was not working was said to lead young men to steal. As Kachieng, a young woman, noted, "If they are not working then you won't expect from them because if they give you they might end up stealing." The same anxiety, as noted in the previous chapter, was shared by older men. Okech noted, for example, "girls give boys huge budgets that makes them to go and steal."[13] Boys were seen as willing to go to great lengths to meet their girlfriends' expectations of provision, regardless of the means or consequences. The onus, then, was on the girlfriend to love her man even if he was poor and not to place huge expectations on him, to have a concurrent relationship with a man who was wealthy, or to leave her poor man so that he would not have to feel frustrated at his inability to provide for her and thus steal.

If girls in sexual relationships felt that their boyfriend had money and was not sharing it with them, then they saw a serious problem. For example, Agnes shared, "I was once having [a boyfriend]. But then I decided to leave him because I was seeing that there is nothing he was helping me with. . . . Like money. He was not even giving me money." She thought that he had money but had chosen not to give her any. So after wondering what was wrong, she decided to just leave him. Her actions were perfectly intelligible to the group of young women among whom she was sharing her experience because the underlying unstated assumption was that money was an expression of love, and therefore he clearly did not love her. In an illustrative moment during a focus group conversation, I asked a group of girls whether a working boyfriend who did not give his girlfriend money was fine with them. Widespread laughter was followed by "you just tell him to quit," "that one is unfaithful," and "he doesn't love you." It was inconceivable to them that a loving man would not share his wealth with his girlfriend. The only explanation would be his miserly nature, his unfaithfulness (and therefore his provision to another woman), or his sheer disregard for her and her family. These were all valid reasons for a girl to leave the man and search for another, not just because he did not help the girl in the short term with whatever things she wanted to buy, but also because it did not bode well for a long-term relationship, where a husband would be expected to provide much more for his wife. A boyfriend with a little money who was willing to share it or who had a willingness to work hard to get the money was a boyfriend with breadwinning, and therefore marriage, potential for the future.

Money was also seen to perform distinct roles within the relationship. One of these was in creating and aiding the growth of love and attachment of girls to male partners. As Leila said in explaining why girls might become sexually active, "someone can go because their parents are poor. And maybe you don't even have clothes, you want to eat these small things and maybe he buys you things like soda. Maybe he buys you a cloth and now you think that this man can be everything for you." Thus, while a girl might not love a man initially and might go to him for explicitly material reasons, his gifts of drink and clothing would lead her to fall in love with him. His own initial display of love and affection, as evidenced by his provision, sparked love and affection in her own mind and heart.

### THE PROBLEM WITH ABSTINENCE
*When Love Is Sex and Sex Is Provision*

These relationship dynamics and others I describe later have interesting implications for thinking about the limits of HIV-prevention effectiveness, especially in longer-term relationships, where HIV transmission is more likely. A strategy often suggested for and by youth was encouraging them to abstain or postpone sexual debut, and knowledge about this prevention strategy was near universal. In the KDHS from 2010, 90% of women and 95% of men cited abstinence as a way to reduce the risk of getting AIDS, and this was reflected in conversations with many of the youth I talked with. They were also clear about how to enact abstinence: as Nancy explained, "you should stick to no with your mouth and with your body." However, this knowledge clashed with the *logic* of relationships. A girl did not become someone's girlfriend unless she had sex with him. As Oyugi, a young man, put it, "sex makes that relationship, it is a complementary unit. Without sex then there is no relationship . . . most of us believe that. Before you engage in sexual intercourse with a girl, then she's not your girlfriend."

In the minds of many young men, sex marked the official start of a relationship where they called a woman their girlfriend. This was partly linked to sex being seen as the ultimate proof of love. As different youth noted "for the love to be called love, sex must be there," that "you find that love cannot last without sex . . . love without sex is like tea without sugar . . . if it's not there, . . . do away with it [the relationship]." If a young man did not eventually approach a young woman he was seeing to ask her for sex, she would think that he did not love her. Eventually, sex had to be there. Indeed, the transition to a relationship for sex was seen as a transition to love. It was a rare woman who was satisfied with a relationship for education. Adam described this dilemma:

> The other thing, when you have a girlfriend, maybe you've not indulged in sex, the lady will keep on asking, "Do you really love me? Do you really love me?" . . . If you say yes, [she will reply,] "how can I know?" The next thing again, "how can I know?" They want you to prove that really you love them. You may buy for them things. Still the question is the same. Do you really love me? Now you say, what again do you need to show that I love you? Surely do you really love me? Now the question keeps on disturbing your mind. If you go to the sex side, maybe you go and do it once, you'll never again have such a question. The next question will be, "nowadays you don't want me." If you don't want to do sex again, the question will be nowadays "you don't want me, you're going to somebody else." But they don't want to tell you "I need sex." No. Nowadays, "you don't love me, you have gone to somebody."

In this excerpt of his response, we see Adam's discussing the pressure from his girlfriend to show love to her. His first strategy is to use words, by telling her he loves her. That is clearly not enough; he has to show it. The next strategy is to "buy for them things." That, however, is still not enough. Sex was necessary to complete the demonstration of love. It is interesting that, rather than directly asking for sex, his girlfriend framed it in terms of how she wanted love expressed. Even after sex began, if he did not have sex with her again, then she might think he was sleeping with somebody else. This in combination with earlier findings suggests that abstinence *or* lack of provision in a relationship meant that there was no proof of love and suspicions of unfaithfulness. This illustrates the entanglement of sex, love, and money as seen in this setting. *Both* sex and money expressed love. In other words, *love = sex + provision*. Thus, really making abstinence work in this setting would require a refashioning of the practice and demonstration of love. Policy strategies such as giving girls money may thus, ironically, place an increased premium on sex as an expression of love.

Further, as noted earlier, engaging in sex was both what ultimately enabled girls to gain access to money and gifts from boyfriends and what in turn encouraged boyfriends to part with hard-earned money. Thus, practicing abstinence among girls meant more than not having sex; it also required self-denial when it came to having what one considered one's *needs* met. Before sex, a young woman could not really have a strong basis for asking her boyfriend for money or gifts. Sex opened the relationship to new claims and requests from her. A young woman would not necessarily see a relationship for sex as a bad thing in practice, unless she had made up her mind to be content with the little she had and to stay away from boys, or unless her parents or family were providing sufficiently (in the girl's mind). This was the case with Clara, for example, who explained that she left her boyfriend even though "he was giving me something," because "I just [saw] that there is no need of it because my parents are still alive and they can really give me those things."

### When Having Sex Means Proving Manhood

Having sex, even if it was "hit-and-run" sex, was also seen by young men and their parents as a way to prove their manhood. (Hit-and-run sex, often occurring in "bush hotels," was the colloquial way youth described a hookup or a one-night stand that happened behind bushes, near local paths throughout the countryside.) Among one group of boys, Kingston said,

> We have so many parents and some of them behave so funny to such an extent that if you see the way some of the parents . . . take their boys, they want them to know . . . their manhood. That, "Okay, this is my boy, is he in a position to [be] staying with a girl?" Those ones are the kinds of things they have to look into. If a parent sees his son has already started getting attracted to some [of] the ladies, he will start saying, "This is my son. I know he will be a very active one. Then I'll be having so many grandchildren."

It was important for parents to see that their sons were showing signs of virility and manhood, and one way of demonstrating this was by having many girlfriends. Platonic relationships did not count. In addition, parents who tried to apply pressure toward abstinence often had no moral ground on which to stand. As one older gentleman, Ochieng, said, "The problem was when parents tried to talk to their kids, the kids would say that parents have done [it] themselves, and now they are old and trying to tell youth to abstain, but how could they abstain? . . . They would say, 'how can you abstain when you are a man? How do you learn that you are a man?'"

Thus, in a setting where being "a man" was measured by success with women, it was hard to tell a young man to abstain, since this was tantamount to telling him to not be a man or to delay his becoming a man and being seen as a man. In a focus group among young men, Harrison described his attempt to abstain and not sleep with his girlfriend, and his subsequent frustrations. "You find that when you're discussing [she may say,] 'You're not a man.' Then you find that a lady is telling you like that, so you have to prove for the lady that you're a man. [Laughter.] So if she tells you like that, you have to go for her." Harrison was describing his experience in high school when he was trying to focus on his schoolwork and pursue a relationship for education. His girlfriend's questioning his manhood, however, prompted him to have sex with her to counter her doubts. He shared this experience in the focus group to make the point that it was not always men who were the aggressors demanding sex in the relationship, but sometimes women. There was no "missing discourse of [young women's] desire in this setting."[14]

In sum, abstinence was not just about not having sex; rather, the *meanings* and expectations attached to sex—love, provision, and masculinity—suggest why knowledge about abstinence for prevention was widespread, but rarely put into practice. Trying to encourage abstinence among youth would rapidly fail if the social underpinning of sex was not taken into account. Asking a young man to abstain would be asking him essentially to not have a girlfriend, to not prove his manhood, and to not prove his love. Asking a young woman to abstain would be asking her to be satisfied with what she had, to cut off her access to gifts and money for her needs, and to limit or postpone her transition to marriage, since for many, a sexual relationship was a prelude to marriage.[15]

TRUST AND CONDOM USE

Another strategy serving as a centerpiece of HIV prevention was urging youth to use condoms. Many youth had clearly received the knowledge: 86% of women and 85% of men in the survey cited condom use as a way to reduce the risk of getting HIV. However, when asked if they used a condom at last sex, 72% of men said yes, but only 24% of women said yes. Part of the reason for this wide gender disparity was marital status—more women in this age group are married than men. Indeed, among the married, 8% of women and 44% of men used a condom at last sex.

This is striking since, even while we might explain married women's low reports of condom use as relating to family building, it is less clear why so many married men in the same age group report condom use, if the same family-building motivation is assumed. This may be one proxy measure of married men's use of condoms with extramarital partners. Among those who had never married, more young people—57% of women and 76% of men—reported condom use at last sex. Even with this increase, however, there are clear gender differences in condom use, with much higher use reported among men, despite young women's much higher HIV risk. Thus, even while awareness of the effectiveness of condoms to reduce risk was equivalent among men and women, the enactment of this prevention strategy clearly varied in gendered ways.

In the interviews, widespread knowledge about condoms (or "CDs," as youth called them) was coupled with widespread discursive ambivalence about condom use, or in some cases outright resistance. Condom use was seen as somewhat paradoxical. As Odhiambo, a young man, put it, "you know when we talk of use of condoms, you know . . . boys and girls . . . involve in sex majorly as a form of pleasure. So you know we believe that condoms will try to hamper with the enjoyment. So if your aim is to feel *yani* [you know] enjoyable and you also use something which is going to hinder that, he will not use it. So . . . boys and girls will object to the use of condoms." Many youth, especially young men, felt that condoms diminished pleasure during sex, and so felt that using one defeated the purpose of sex. As a result, they said it was better to tell them to abstain than to tell them to use a condom. Further, as has been similarly observed in other settings, condoms were likened to eating bananas with the peels on or eating a sweet still in the plastic wrapping. People preferred *nyama kwa nyama*, or flesh against flesh. These phrases and sayings were recited in almost every setting where the subject of condoms was brought up.[16]

Perhaps the real reason underlying high school boys' resistance, however, was their limited opportunities to have sex. Several school-going males discussed their concern about the period between convincing a girl to sleep with them and finding and putting on a condom. Mark gave a typical description in a focus group of this anxiety:

> You know some of the boys will be thinking that for all that long that I'll be taking, putting on this condom, maybe, she might even change her mind. *[Laughter.]* She might even change her mind and then decide to leave. Then what do I do? Then whatever happens is, let me just do this thing and put everything to God. *[Laughter.]* And actually after doing that thing, that's when your eyes will be opened, wide open and then you will start thinking . . . now what did I do? Have I already contracted this HIV/AIDS? That's where the problem lies.

As discussed earlier, for a young man to bring a young woman to the point of agreeing to have sex with him was a big deal. It was likely to be a relatively rare, sometimes one-time event. Jeopardizing this prime opportunity for the sake of a condom that would diminish their pleasure was hard for young men to conceive. The fear that their girlfriend would change her mind was even more real for young men in light of what they thought would be their girlfriend's reaction if they used a condom. The survey data shows that condom use increased with age. For young men, this was perhaps the result of increased experience with condoms and sex; as they got older, increasing resources made them more attractive sexual partners, thus providing more opportunities to have sex. Therefore, they had less to lose if their partner changed her mind if they used a condom. Additionally, their experience with the HIV epidemic and AIDS mortality would also cumulate as they aged, perhaps giving them increased incentive to use condoms.[17]

Both young men and women said in interviews that they thought the highest-risk age group for AIDS was their own; those were the people they saw dying. Many did not expect their partners to be faithful, and, as the survey results support, many knew that condoms or abstinence were the only way in which they could prevent themselves from getting it. Given these understandings, it is surprising that, especially among women, condom use was not higher. Many arguments in the literature suggest, with some justification, that while young women have agency in entering and exiting relationships, they have little agency when it comes to negotiating safe sex. This is arguably further undermined by the power imbalances introduced by the exchange of money within relationships. This would be a key explanation for the 19-percentage-point disparity between men's and women's reports of condom use. However, these arguments assume that young women *want* to negotiate safe sex, and would if they could. In other words, the assumptions are that "men and women have different preferences for risky sexual behavior. The male partner prefers unsafe sexual activities, such as unprotected sex (the nonuse of condoms and contraception), and the female prefers safe behavior."[18] However, in this setting, there were reasons that belied this understanding. Some men, for example, described how wanting to use a condom might make their girlfriends think their boyfriends saw them as prostitutes. In an argument Janet overheard between a man and woman, the woman said, "You think I'm a prostitute? Why do you want to use a condom on me? If you don't trust me, then go." Further, in the course of a relationship, the use of a condom became increasingly difficult. After a young woman had agreed to allow a young man to have sex with her, for him to ask her to use a condom was difficult; indeed, the continued use of condoms was an insult. In Peter's words, "From my experience, you can't use a condom for three consecutive times with your girlfriend. Because she will say you don't trust her. [She will say,] 'You think I have AIDS.' For the first time you can use it, and for the second time, but for the third time if you are still continuing with it then she will force you to leave it. So I think condoms can only be used successfully in the cases of hit and run."

From men's point of view, then, it was not just men who didn't want to use condoms, but also women, especially in the context of a relationship. Condoms might be useful and acceptable for the one-night stands, but not for long-term relationships.[19] The gender disparity in condom use might thus reflect the reality that young men had a greater likelihood of being in one-night stands and, therefore, of using condoms, while young women had a greater likelihood of being in longer-term relationships where condoms had been abandoned. The problem, of course, because of the epidemiology of HIV transmission noted earlier, is that the danger lies in long-term concurrent relationships rather than one-off sexual encounters,[20] even though some condom use was better than nothing. Shelley Clark and her colleagues found that among young people in Kisumu, Nyanza, relationships headed toward marriage were in fact less likely to involve condom use.[21] Further underscoring the relationship logics in this setting, Nancy Luke and colleagues, using the same data, found that the more monetary or gift transfers young women received, the more likely they were to engage in sex, and the less likely they were to use condoms.[22] More financial support suggested more investment in the relationship on the part of men. Less condom use, in turn, suggested trust on the part of women. Thus, in contexts where "safe" sex is conceived of as a lack of trust within a sexual relationship, especially if the young women were attempting to convert the relationship into something more permanent through pregnancy, clearly these assumptions do not hold up. "Trust," for many young women, was their "prophylactic strategy."[23] Indeed, in a context where AIDS was so ubiquitous that it had become part of the regular relationship dialogue—"you think I have AIDS?"—*not* using a condom was a performance of trust and even love. Women, in perhaps the ultimate act of love, were quite literally putting their life in the hands of their man. Ironically, then, young people were more likely to use condoms in the *least risky* relationships—one-night stands and hit and runs—and to abandon them in their *most serious* relationships. Perhaps one of the most tragic things about HIV is that it is often received from the person whom one loves the most.

## GENDER AND MONEY

In thinking through the relationship logics in this setting, money clearly played a central role in the debut, progression, maintenance, and ending of sexual relationships among young people. However, it clearly meant and played different roles for men and women. In this next section, I delve deeper into examining gender differences in the meaning and importance of money and male provision, and how these differences are linked to the last centerpiece of HIV prevention, limiting concurrency and being faithful.

### Money and Masculinity

In truth, many young men were broke, and making ends meet, especially in the early years after receiving an education, was a constant struggle. Reflecting this reality, young men's discussions about relationships were often characterized by bitterness, primarily stemming from their belief that their lack of money stood in the way of ideal relationships. Men in relationships or in search of them clearly saw themselves cast in a role of "provider" that they could not yet comfortably fulfill, and they were often frustrated because of it. In one conversation with a group of young men, for example, I asked them whether girlfriends were expensive to have, and Jimmy responded, "I had a girlfriend. She was very expensive in that she will need always sanitary towels [pads], oils that will make her comfortable, and some clothes that [I could not] afford, so having a girlfriend [was] just a problem and very expensive . . . the relationship couldn't have continued if I couldn't provide."

As a result, many young men felt that they lost out to sugar daddies and men who were working and had money. Indeed, it sometimes seemed as if the main reason boys wanted money was so that they could have a girlfriend. As Omondi put it, "We need more than girls because everything that girls can need, they get three-quarters from us." What was left unstated was the fact that young men were having to provide in the face of young women's fathers' inability to provide financially in a context of widespread poverty and many mouths to feed in a household, fathers who were absent because they had migrated for work and were not sending regular remittances home, or fathers who had passed away.

Money was helpful in starting relationships, because it demonstrated to a prospective girlfriend that a man was worth having. John put it this way:

> You know men, they want to be recognized, you see. So me as a young person, I want people to recognize who I am. So I'm approaching ladies. So you find sometimes I'm not capable with my speeching. You see I cannot . . . convince, so I'll have to use money. So by using money, it is men giving out money, not ladies to go out and work for money. But because men . . . don't have that ability to convince, they are using money to at least convince one or two. So that one will prove that they are men.

Money was needed to prove manhood, which it did by impressing women and paving the way for a successful proposition to a young woman. It helped a man surmount his shortcomings and stood in for his lack of eloquence in chatting up a woman. Money was seen to speak louder than or in place of words. The audience, however, was not just the young woman in question, but those witnessing his largesse and attractiveness to women. He would be "recognized" even if he was a young person.

Money, as noted earlier, was also needed to maintain relationships, especially once a relationship began to involve sex. For boys to show their love, they had to help their girlfriends, and helping often involved working to make money to give to their girlfriends. At the conclusion of a couple of interviews at a remote school in one of the study districts, I hired a bicycle-taxi *(boda boda)* young man for transportation back to the main road where I could catch a *matatu* back to the main town. On my arrival back to my lodging several hours later, I recorded the following reflective field note:

> The *boda boda* guy on the way back was also a Standard 8 [primary school graduate] who didn't have money for secondary. He said that he makes

about Kshs 150 ($2) on a good day, especially when there are funerals and lots of people heading up. He said there was one coming up on Friday. He said that there weren't any jobs for girls to do, except perhaps collecting firewood from the hills (the hills looked really really far away) and selling them. Other than that they were completely dependent on parents. He said it was hard for them to get money. There were no girls doing this bike work I noticed; just a stable of mainly young boys and a few older ones. There were two men who passed by pushing/pulling a *mabati mkokoteni* [corrugated iron-wheel barrow] with large logs of wood. He said that they could be paid about Kshs 400 ($5) for the job—delivering the wood from a town about 15 km away to near where the school was. And sometimes the *mkokoteni* was also hired, so the owner would want Kshs 100/day for the hire [of the wheelbarrow]. And they had to return it [that is, walk it 15 km back]. And sometimes that could be the only job of the day. So a lot of work for little money. One of the boys yesterday said that to get money they have to sweat for it. It's not easy. No wonder they are reluctant to give it to girls for nothing.

Many young men, in conversations, had seemed deeply resentful of the predicament they found themselves in: having to sweat and work hard for little money, and then give it away to girlfriends. Observing this sweating and the many hard hours young men put in for their money made sense of their reactions.

As if to further underscore poor young men's challenges, there was a sense that the male provision of money was a prerequisite not just for a relationship for sex, but also for a *faithful* relationship.[24] For example, when I asked Preston, "So you don't think that boys can have a girlfriend if they don't have a job or don't have money?" he responded, " I think you can have but this girl will just be your girlfriend and then she will be looking for money somewhere so she can bring you a disease." Concurrency was felt to be more likely if a man did not have money. If he could not afford to provide for his girlfriend, and she chose to remain his girlfriend, then it was understood that she might have to search for money from another man.

### AVOIDING HIV

It was precisely *because* of the entanglement of money with relationships for sex that young men with no money also inadvertently avoided HIV.

For young men who wanted to pursue relationships, many chose to avoid girls they perceived as expensive or financially demanding, even though they recognized that these expenses were spent on products to make them look beautiful and attractive. For example, one young man out of school, Jack, noted in a focus group:

> The lives of girls are more expensive than those of men. You find that she wants to lead the same life as maybe a friend or even a cousin is living. Maybe yourself you can't afford but she forces you. So maybe you will say no, that is too much for me, you can just leave.

Tom, also a young man out of school, followed:

> To add on to that, I think that you may want a girl, but if she is willing to be the way you are, then you will start at that and rise slowly. But then if she doesn't want then you will just say this is wrong number, then leave her.

Many young men started out relatively poor when they left school. Work life often began with itinerant low-paying jobs such as bicycle-taxi work. (I discuss youth employment in chapter 6.) In this situation, pursuing relationships involved deciding whether they could afford the woman they were attracted to. For those wanting relationships, in exercising the choice to avoid expensive women and instead selecting girls who were "willing to be the way they were," they were essentially choosing young women who had low consumption needs—girls who were not consuming women—and who were less likely to expect provision and less likely to pursue concurrent relationships. Relationships characterized by fewer material transfers were also less likely to involve sex,[25] and there was thus less exposure to HIV.

Other young men framed spending money on young women as a waste, and therefore avoided relationships altogether. For example, Obongo, a young man, said:

> There's this provincial ball games, so most of us went. That is why even the [school] population is a bit low. And when they go, me I remain, because I don't see the need of wasting money there. Going and then cheating a girl that I love her, that she's the only one and then when I come back here again, when I go home I also see another and say, you know, "you're the only one." So it does not interest me, so I said no. I prioritize things in my life and I

took it as my responsibility to either make a future for myself or destroy a future for myself.

In this excerpt, Obongo was describing his conscious decision not to "waste" his money on girls at the large sports festival drawing students of both genders from across the province. For most schoolboys, this would be a prime opportunity to meet girls; however, it would also be an expensive event, since they would have to spend money buying things to impress and win over the girls they were meeting, along with saying the magic words "I love you." He, however, had chosen to remain in school and focus on his schoolwork. Another way of viewing this attitude of some young men, however, is that they were simply trying to find a way to reconcile themselves to the fact that they were not young women's preferred partners, at least for now. Rather than dealing with constant rejection and failure or "wasting money" on relationships that were not going to last, they preferred to be satisfied with relationships for education or to simply work toward gaining the future status that would allow them to be a success on the playing field of relationships in a few years. In this way, young men's low HIV-prevalence rates reflected a combination of inadvertently protective strategies. Substantial numbers of young men were either rejecting or postponing sexual relationships, engaging in occasional hit-and-run sex, or choosing nonconsuming women as partners.

## MONEY, WOMEN, AND TRANSACTIONAL RELATIONSHIPS

### Transactional Relationships and Community Ambivalence

Voicing out loud what many other young men were no doubt thinking about the young women they encountered in their everyday lives, Humphrey commented, "the kind of dresses they are putting on, they lure so much. In that, you can be tempted. So many men are tempted." Male standards of beauty had dramatically changed over the twentieth century, as discussed in chapter 3. Now, Luo men assessed beauty based on skin shade, makeup, and how dressed up a woman was. However, modern dresses, skin creams, and makeup had to be bought. Ideal desirable women, in other words, had to be *consuming* women, women whose "lives

were expensive." Their wanting and needing money were thus in many
ways a response to changing male standards of beauty and taste. Despite
young men's complaints about young women's extravagant and expensive
needs (as elaborated earlier), it was nonetheless true that everyone in Luo
land admired a well-dressed, well-made-up young woman. In many towns
and villages across the province, men would frequently and openly com-
pliment young women on their beauty and appearance, and proposition
them in public places and on public transportation vehicles. While young
women would give the impression of embarrassment, shyness, and even
irritation, they often did not turn these men away. It was not always clear
in observing these interactions whether young women experienced them
as complimentary, as public harassment, or both. There was an implicit
understanding among all concerned of the relatively high expense of
dressing well and looking good among a group of young women everyone
knew could not afford to maintain themselves on their own income.
Consuming women either came from a wealthy family or were being supported by someone who was earning an income. Young women's consumption needs made sense in a context where goods-enhanced beauty
was valorized, and where boyfriends' money was put toward the discipline
of making themselves into ideal desirable women whom their boyfriends,
and boyfriends' friends and parents, could appreciate. However, although
such young women were admired, there was considerable ambivalence
about their means of acquiring the money to become admirable.

In the community, contradictions abounded in discussions of young
women's transactional relationships (but interestingly, not about their male
partners). Condemnation of these relationships was widespread, from out-
raged public officials to key informants to local community members. Yet, it
was apparent that there was tacit approval in practice. Mrs. Ojwang, a
teacher, for example, described the attitude of parents in her community:
"[They believe that] once a girl has reached the age of 12, [she] can now
take care of [her]self. So . . . if they go asking for something like sanitary
towels [pads], they are told, 'You're now a big girl, you can get this one on
your own.' So when they've been told like that, they go ahead looking for it
where they can get it. And the only source is now selling themselves to men
. . . that's the only source of income. Apart from parents, now only boyfriends." The ambivalence felt about these relationships is apparent in the

quotation; even while the teacher uses the language of commercial sex, saying that girls are "selling themselves," we also see her using the language of
romance, for example, when she says "now only boyfriends" instead of "male
clients." In another conversation recorded in a field note, a community
health worker described how: "when a girl goes out at night and comes back
the following morning bringing Blue Band [a type of margarine], bread,
and so on, instead of rebuking her or asking the daughter where she got
those things, a mother would be delighted, and excited saying, 'Kawuono
wabiro chiemo maber!' [Today we're going to eat well!]." Thus, it was not
always clear that in practice these relationships were truly considered deviant, if they accomplished valued ends such as good food (as breakfast foods
went, bread and margarine were a step up from grain-based porridge [such
as millet or oats porridge] or maize and beans).[26]

Parents were in a difficult situation because of their financial hardships
and their inability to provide for their children beyond the basic provision
of food and shelter. In communities where stark and relative poverty coex-
isted with small pools of wealth, a daughter's boyfriend who was willing to
share his resources and bring small improvements to everyday life in order
to bolster her family was seen as welcome support. Thus, in some cases,
parents would explicitly encourage their daughters, as the following discussion in a focus group of schoolgirls illustrated:

PRISCILLA: Even in the case where you have both parents, let's say that they are
alive, both of them but they doesn't have any work which they can
do in order to provide your needs. So they will not even bother you
a lot because so long as you can provide those things by yourself,
you will not come to them asking them for them. So they can just
leave you anyhow to go and look for them.

SANYU: So you think part of the problem is parents don't have enough money
to support the children?

HELEN: But now madam, some parents do encourage this issue. Let's take a
house where all the parents are poor, you know even a mother can
go and tell her girl, "you just go and have even a boyfriend so whenever he gives you something, you come back to the house and we
share." That is the case.[27]

Other families would simply have a "don't ask, don't tell" policy, as another
school girl, Dorica, noted, "You know maybe you can tell your father . . .

you are entering into matters which you're not supposed to enter [or it's not appropriate for you to enter]. I am sure even you [referring to Sanyu], the way you are, your father cannot ask you everything. Even if you buy your panties these days, will he ask you where you got it?" Thus, while the ends were valued, and even encouraged by some parents, few wanted to know the means by which those ends were accomplished. This makes sense of why girls would be surreptitious about the way they went about their relationships, as I discuss in the next section.[28]

Receiving money and gifts also served longer-term goals for young women. A boyfriend's provision of money and gifts helped her to become a desirable woman capable of attracting a husband who could maintain her in that style, whether or not her current boyfriend was "the one." However, his provision of money and gifts could also be a sign to a young woman that he was in fact "the one." His gifts were not only demonstrating his love for her through sometimes sacrificial giving; he was also demonstrating his ability and willingness to provide for her and her family, and thus his long-term suitability as a husband. Ironically, it was in relationships with men who could *continually* provide and therefore sustain a longer-term sexual relationship that young women were at the greatest risk for acquiring HIV.[29] As noted earlier, the low probability of acquiring HIV through a single encounter suggests that young women were more likely to get HIV from these sorts of longer-term relationships than short-term relationships. The riskiest relationships, thus, were either in marriage or through transactional relationships with older men who could continually provide. I turn to examining these relationships next.

*Money and Unmarried Young Women's Relationships
with Older Men*

As noted earlier, the survey data suggest that a substantial proportion of unmarried teenagers' risk came from relationships with unmarried men in their early 20s or married men. For both sets of older men—those married and unmarried—the key factor was their ability to provide. The more consumption needs or desires a young woman had, the more likely it was that one of her sexual partners was a wealthy man and thus potentially older than her by several years, and working with regular access to money.

Young women's preferred partners seemed predominantly to be men in the community who worked or were salaried with access to steady income. They called these men "working-class" men. Thus, it was not so much age that determined the type of partners they chose, but rather men's access to income and their willingness to share it with them. Categorized this way, several men were only a few years older, in their early to mid-20s. In a study in Kisumu, only 5% of Luo men self-reported as having partners 10 or more years younger than themselves, a much lower prevalence than popular perceptions suggest. However, 70% of men's partnerships were with women five or more years younger.[30] In terms of HIV risk, as figure 11 suggests, this age difference was sufficient for young women's high risk.

Many of these men for girls in communities near the lake were fishermen, fairly young men in their mid- to late 20s, but with daily access to money (from the sale of fish every morning), who would have relationships with girls and support them with money. Others were bank managers who might give them as much as Kshs 2000 ($28) at a time, others were *boda boda* (bicycle taxi) men and day laborers, who gave much less money (Kshs 50 [$.71]) during the course of their relationship. Construction crew members building roads through various communities were more explicitly temporary partners, since once that part of the road was built, the men would move on to another community and new sets of women and girls. Other men described were older men ("they have got some wrinkles"), married men, and men who sponsored young women through school. While some of these men lived in their community, many were also married migrant workers who came home to visit family periodically. While the processual nature of dating relationships among young women meant that it was not always clear whether they would be converted into permanent long-term relationships or would end, the possibility of marriage as a first or secondary wife was left open in their minds. However, whenever young women talked about sexual relationships with men considerably older than themselves, marriage was rarely a stated intention.[31] They wanted to marry men their own age or slightly older. When asked, ideal age differences ranged from two to four years older. In terms of ideals, then, relationships with older men were more explicitly short term in young women's minds than those with men of a similar age, who were poorer but had a long-term potential of one day being financially able.[32]

A sugar daddy was often found in clubs. Thus, a girl wanting to find one would "have to leave home when your parents don't know. . . . You sneak at night, go to the clubs, then you will find a sugar daddy there, then you will be there dancing very nicely, and the sugar daddy was comforting himself with a soda, and the moment he sees you dancing very nicely, he just sends another person to call that girl, that is the way you will engage yourself with that man." Clubs in Luo land were popular places for men to go after work and hang out with their friends. In such settings, roasted meat and fish would be washed down with soda or beer, while local musicians played the *nyatiti*, or acoustic guitar, and sang Luo music. A typical evening would end with dancing. Away from their wives, and in the presence of approving middle-aged peers, clubs presented an ideal place for them to discreetly pick up younger girlfriends.[33]

There were many reasons girls gave for why sugar daddies were preferable to same-aged boyfriends who were, epidemiologically speaking, almost risk free. For one thing, sugar daddies simply had more money. Okello, a young man, complained, "And now because girls have known that most boys who are students don't have money, they go to sugar daddies to give them money." Most young men going to school could not afford to compete with sugar daddies in this way. Those out of school would also not be earning enough both to cater to their needs and to give money to a young woman until they had been working for a few years. So they were also shut out. Another factor was that, as men who worked, sugar daddies were conveniently distant. Maggie elaborated:

> Mostly people choose sugar daddies, because the boyfriends, you know they give people more stress. . . . They will be watching your every move. . . . With them they will be always near where you are, even in the estate [urban residential communities], they will be seeing you but sugar daddies, daytime they are at work but the boys, at daytime they will be at home, so if you attempt to talk to another boy, or make a relationship with another boy, he will see you and the fight will start. But the sugar daddy will only see you at night or weekends or in the clubs.

Further, the sugar daddy demanded neither love nor faithfulness. Girls noted how "the sugar daddy will not mind even if you don't love him," and how "they will not bother even if you tell them that that was my brother but the boys, they will know." Young women liked the freedom that relationships with sugar daddies gave them, feeling that their same-aged counterparts were too possessive and too demanding. This freedom was particularly valuable for young women who were still in school or who had temporarily dropped out but still anticipated returning to school.[34] They were not ready to get married, since marriage, in this setting, meant the end of school. However, having such a relationship would allow them to have money to buy their "small small" things while their parents focused on finding money for school expenses or money to feed the household. A pretty bar of soap or a bottle of perfume would not rank high on many families' lists of needs. Meanwhile, young women would also be able to pursue a "relationship for education" with a schoolboy they really liked, but who was comparatively poor. Both relationships would place little by way of emotional demands on a teenage girl. By contrast, a relationship for sex with a boyfriend her own age would bring not only "stress," but also little by way of financial benefit. Finally, girls found that the sex and, in some cases, the emotional quality of the relationship was better with older men.[35] An older gentleman, Ogugi, had been puzzling over why a young woman he was trying to mentor was always having relationships with older men. Her answer was simple: "A young man can jump on you eight times in the night and you are not satisfied. An old man can jump on you once, and you will even be satisfied for a month." Compared to young men, older men had many more years of sexual experience and thus were better able to meet the needs of young women just beginning their sex lives.

All these reasons, then, suggest that a young woman's relationship with an older man would be even more dangerous in an epidemiological sense. This setup allowed such relationships with older men who had high HIV rates to persist for a longer period of time than a relationship for sex with a same-aged boyfriend through a combination of considerably better financial support especially before marriage, better sex, and freedom from emotional demands. This freedom ironically made these relationships perfectly compatible with pursuing education. Thus, being a modern young woman who went to school and consumed meant pursuing a relationship with a providing man who was also more likely to be a high-risk partner, while avoiding a stressful and poor same-aged partner.

*Money and Marriage*

In contemporary times, marriage was increasingly less likely to be characterized by the elaborate process described in chapter 3. In the more common transition to marriage, a couple typically moved in together in cohabiting relationships colloquially called "come we stay," and eventually, perhaps after a child or two, the man might bring a cow to the girl's family, or not, as was often the case. Formal introduction ceremonies could happen long after the beginning of cohabitation, and any gift to the family was a mere token compared to the amount a man might have been expected to pay in the past. These changes no doubt reflect the changing socioeconomy, with fewer men able to afford the cost of "traditional" marriage.[36] It was perhaps because of this that men who could afford it were considered more attractive husbands in the eyes of the girl's family. In this way, money was entangled in marital decisions in ways that sometimes overrode purely romantic considerations, even though marriage was largely considered young women's choice. Marriage continued to be seen by a family as a major way in which they could obtain wealth to help feed the family, to educate younger siblings, and to help provide bride wealth for sons in the family wanting to get married. Girls were particularly vulnerable to quick or unexpected marriages if there was no money for school fees or if she was out of school and her family was poor. They were then "forced by circumstances" to get married, "because you may find that even there are some parents who cannot look after you so [you] decide to go." This was especially true for orphan girls. For example Jenny, now 23, described how, while she was able to finish high school, she lost first her mother and then her father within a year of each other. At that point, her dream of going on to study business administration in college was no longer possible, and she saw herself as having no options. She said that she and a lot of orphan girls had no choice but to get married "if you are desperate." Her two siblings stayed with her grandmother as she established her marital household. Her story was particularly hopeful in that her husband sponsored her for a course that enabled her to subsequently establish an independent business.

A daughter's husband became an additional source of income for a family. They could periodically ask a daughter to send them money from her household budget to help with her siblings' expenses, especially before she had her own children. Families could also send a sibling to go and live with a married sister to reduce the costs on the natal household. Thus, if a rich suitor came asking for their daughter, "they have to accept because he is rich, so [even if] the girl is young, they just accept." Unlike many young men with whom a young woman might go and live and thus informally "marry," a rich man could afford to give considerable gifts in the form of food, animals (for example, cattle or goats), and cash to the girl's family, and could contract a proper marriage based on bride wealth. Consequently, such suitors were preferable to parents.[37]

Given their wealth, these men were likely to be much older than the girls and, in some cases, also polygamous. Young women would thus often become a second or third wife. One in five women (23%) under 30 years of age were in polygamous marriages in this setting, compared to only 3.5% of same-aged men. (As noted in chapter 3, a quarter of men over 30 had more than one wife.) This supports the sense that many young women were in highly risky marriages. Not only were they married to husbands in an age category of high risk, but also their risk of encountering HIV had increased. One infected wife or husband in such a partnership could transmit HIV to all members of the marriage. This would also have the effect of contributing to wide gendered disparities in HIV rates among young people.

Money continued to be important to women even after they were married, not just to support their natal families, but also for their own continued consumption. Having been attracted by consuming women, Luo men would work hard to help their wives continue to purchase desirability and meet cultural standards of beauty. The following field note, a summary of an extended conversation I had with a middle-aged gentleman, Omondi, his female secretary Amollo, and my research assistant Marian, all Luo, illustrates this well:

> Discussing modern Luo marriages, Omondi described how Luo ladies would want their man in charge—i.e. take care of all the bills and so on, leaving the Luo lady to just think about her wardrobe (dressing), her hair, and maybe money to send to her parents. After he said this, Amollo and Marian who I was with in the room burst out laughing and continued to do so for a long time saying, "it is true, it is true." He went on to talk about special

occasions where a lady would not wear the same outfit again. She needed to have a different outfit for each occasion. So the man should not put a lot of strain on her income, and should not budget for the home using all her income. I asked whether he was saying Luo ladies were expensive to maintain, and he agreed, as did the ladies. He added that as a man, he should take care of household expenses and leave her to spend her money. Once in a while, he should buy her a dress, and choose carefully, paying careful attention to the colors. He said on a side note that even *mitumbas* [second-hand clothes sellers] in Nyanza knew there were certain colors they did not sell in Nyanza because they just would not sell. The Luo were particular about such things. That, he said, is how the Luo are; income is the only restraint or thing holding them back from how they would like to live. This is the ideal they strive for, in other words. Luo like good things.

This description of ideal household dynamics and expectations between a Luo husband and his wife illustrates the continued expectation after marriage of a man's provision above and beyond basic needs. To the extent that a man was able, providing for a wife's consumption was a valued attribute. This gives a picture of the kind of characteristics an unmarried young woman might be looking to be demonstrated in a potential mate, and the expectations a married woman might place on her husband, key among which is a man who was generous and could provide good things for her beyond household basic needs. In other words, similar to dynamics described in chapter 2, marital relationships were expected to be lovingly nourished by men through consumption and codified in purchased products such as clothing.

## "FAITHFULNESS . . . DOES NOT CONCUR WITH THE MIND"

Another key pillar of HIV-prevention strategies is faithfulness. In the survey, 93% of women and 92% of men cited having only one partner as a way to reduce the risk of getting AIDS. However, as illustrated in this chapter, it is not just married men who were having extramarital affairs, but also many young unmarried women who had married male partners. With this information, the survey demonstrated that knowledge was apparently not reflected in behavioral reality. Precisely the kinds of men who could afford to marry—working-class men, breadwinners—were the kinds of men most able to sustain providing relationships with extramarital partners. The high HIV-prevalence levels in this setting mean that even serial monogamy and a faithful partnership in the course of that relationship could be risky. However, concurrency was clearly a factor in this setting. Indeed, there seemed to be a belief engrained in the minds of everyone I talked with that Luo men could not be faithful.[38] For Christopher, the idea was incredulous. "Matters pertaining to faithfulness, actually you know, it does not concur with the mind." Men needed a "balanced diet" since "maybe sometimes he is bored up with the daily meal he used to take [and] he wants to change diet." They did not believe men could be faithful either before or even after marriage. Luo women invariably shared this perception. The only exception in my interviews and conversations was men characterized as serious Christians and saved, and these men were seen as rare or "about 1%." Encapsulating this perspective, Linda noted that a husband's faithfulness "can be possible. You can be a God-loving girl and maybe you are saved and you can go and counsel your husband. Whether he was saved or not saved, it is you who can change the life of that husband. So you can just, after being saved, you can [both] be faithful in your home."[39]

While the idea of men's faithfulness seemed unnatural or inconceivable, women's faithfulness, for many, was determined by circumstances and was conditional on whether they had what they *materially* needed.[40] In a conversation with a group of young women, for example, Anyango noted, "Women are the most faithful people . . . only if they are being provided with what they will need. . . . The woman, she will go to another man if the husband is not providing with the needs. So she may go even to another man to provide with . . . basic needs. Maybe you have children. They lack basic needs, so you just go." The understanding was that if a man could not provide, and a woman's own resources did not stretch far enough, then a concurrent partnership with a man who could provide was seen as a viable and understandable option. Similarly, in this fashion, unmarried girls whose needs were not met could justify concurrent relationships with their poor school boyfriend for education and with a working-class man who could provide. As I will argue in the next chapter, it was what counted as "basic needs" that ultimately motivated transactional relationships.

## HIV TESTING AND STATUS AWARENESS

Constructing ABC as impossible and unrealistic resulted in youth throwing their hands in the air. In an expression of this, Crispa, a young woman, remarked to much laughter, "if people can't abstain and they can't use condoms, so let us just pray."[41] However, a strategy that increasing numbers of young people were pursuing was making a conscious choice to engage in HIV testing and awareness, to know their HIV status, and thus to keep themselves and others safe.

There were high rates of personal HIV status awareness among Luo-Nyanza youth. In the KDHS from 2010, among teenagers, 50% of women and 42% of men had ever been tested for HIV. Among 20–24 year olds, 82% and 84% of women and men, respectively, had been tested.[42] Of those who tested HIV positive among teenagers, fewer girls (75%) than boys (88%) had been tested. However, for 20–24 year olds, slightly more women (87%) than men (73%) had been tested. In all cases, there was nearly universal receipt of results, indicating that many young people who were HIV positive likely knew it.[43] These findings represent a dramatic improvement in HIV testing and awareness between the DHS survey in 2004 and 2010. Only 33% of teenage girls who were HIV positive then, for example, knew their status. The key factor accounting for higher HIV testing was the mass rollout of antiretroviral (ARV) medication, which I observed taking root during fieldwork, and its being made available for free in communities across Nyanza. This might also underlie, to some extent, high HIV-prevalence levels among youth in their 20s and above who might otherwise have died of HIV, but are now gaining access to ARV medication. However, despite high rates of awareness of personal HIV status, rates among teenage boys and girls have *tripled* since 2004 (as noted at the beginning of the chapter) and reflect less survival and more new acquisition of HIV.[44] This suggests a continued gap between HIV/AIDS-prevention knowledge, HIV-status awareness, and relationship practices. HIV testing, when it was occurring, was for information, not prevention.

There were clear variations in the use of HIV testing based on relationship status. HIV testing was much higher among those who married. Much higher proportions of married women had been tested compared to women who had never married. Among 15–19 year olds, 91% of married and 40% of unmarried teenagers had ever been tested. Among 20–24 year olds, 81% of married and 67% of unmarried young women had ever been tested. This was both because many women were likely to have been tested as part of their antenatal screenings,[45] and because testing was beginning to be used among those planning to marry. Caroline Kabiru and colleagues, studying youth in the capital Kisumu, found that women who wanted to marry had almost twice the odds (OR 1.73) of having an HIV test compared to those who did not wish to marry. The findings were not, however, significant for men. They also found that men (but not women) in concurrent relationships were more likely (OR 3.2) to have had an HIV test, suggesting that men, in another example of "knowing but ignoring," were fully aware of the risk they were engaging in by having multiple partners.[46] The interesting picture that emerges from the study is that women got a test if they were intending to marry, but not if they were in a concurrent relationship. However, men got a test in concurrent relationships, but not if they were intending to marry. This suggests that HIV-status checks were important markers of women's marital suitability but not of men's and, further, that the gender disparity in premarital HIV testing may have reflected a lack of volition in women's testing practices. That is, while men know their partners' status, women do not. Indeed, research suggests that knowing one's HIV-negative status can result in riskier, not safer, behavior, as the men's actions in this study suggest.[47]

The outcome of a test could sometimes be heartbreaking for a couple, as the following excerpt from an interview with an HIV-positive young woman, Mara, illustrates:

MARA:   I went for the [HIV] test and found I was positive. When I went to tell my partner, he complained a lot and we decided to go for the test together. He came out negative but for me I was positive and from then he isn't that close to me.

SANYU:   How did you meet?

MARA:   He came to my house to ask for the relationship. He isn't in school. He is just working and is 24.

Mara had only had two sexual partners: her high school–going boyfriend, the father of her first child, from whom she thinks she contracted HIV,

and her current partner, the father of her second child. She had been living with HIV for possibly as long as six years. Knowing her HIV status
was, for her, a mixed blessing. It, along with the existence of ARVs in her
community for free, gave her a hopeful outlook on life. AIDS was no
longer a death sentence, and she could envisage a future watching her
sons grow up while running her small business. However, it had also given
her current partner pause. They were now part of the millions of HIV
sero-discordant couples in Africa,[48] and his knowledge of his negative
HIV status and his partner's positive HIV status had made him pull away.
The early age of cohabitation and marriage in this community means that
this scenario was likely typical of the discovery of an HIV-positive status
among young women, since their rates were much higher than same-aged
men. Many young women were likely in the same place as Mara, acquiring
HIV in their teens, getting into long-term relationships, and discovering
this reality early after their first pregnancy or the birth of their first or
second child. Many have the conjoined and painful discovery of sex, love,
and a life partner alongside a life-altering HIV diagnosis. For young men
like Mara's partner, knowing his and his partner's HIV status had led to
his distancing himself from her, thus breaking her heart, but limiting his
own exposure to HIV.

CONCLUSION

Youth in Luo-Nyanza were navigating their romantic lives in a context of
high HIV prevalence. Young Luo women were caught in the middle,
between their trying to become the well-dressed and desirable women
most admired in their community (inadvertently consuming women),
their own financial limitations in the face of these needs and desires, and
their longing to find working or well-off husbands. Their sexual relationships were contexts within which care and love were expressed through
money and gifts, gifts that in turn helped them meet Luo ideals of beauty
and ideal womanhood—dressing well and looking good. However, their
relationship choices were not driven by the need to avoid HIV. Rather,
they were driven by a romantic system in which love, sex, and money were
entangled, and in which the logic of relationships led young women to

choose the highest-risk partners—men who could show love through provision—and resulted in young men only being able to afford the lowest-risk partners or no partners at all.

Above and beyond young women's individual choices, however, their actions and motivations were also clearly shaped by social structure. As we have seen, community norms, value systems, and collective practices played an important role in shaping the context, cultural scripts, and logics through which young women pursued and made sense of their relationships. In the next chapter, I examine the social structure of school, and show how young women's needs and desires, which we have seen were expressed and met in the context of relationships, are in fact cultivated in school. More, I illustrate how school, in a similar way to communities, inadvertently *produced* consuming women and made it impossible for some young women to both pursue education and stay safe from HIV risk.

# 5 School and the Production of Consuming Women

A joke with a man is a child or a disease.

A father, to his school-going daughter

For many young women, completing a high school education without getting pregnant or contracting HIV was an anomaly and was tied in important ways to the role of consumption and money in romantic relationships. In this chapter, I will explore in greater depth the role of school in complicating young women's attempts to stay HIV free. I first begin by describing the complicated relationship between education and HIV in the literature, before discussing the rise and popularity of mass education as a means for social mobility in Kenya, and its role in creating modern subjects. The chapter will then focus on examining how school structures HIV risk. I examine how school produces consuming women by examining the language of "needs" used by men and women in the previous chapter. I show how school exacerbates gendered needs in ways that produce gendered consumer desires. I then discuss the challenges of negotiating the school environment, and I also consider the competing normative systems young women were navigating. Finally I examine the consequences of high teacher mortality rates for young women's HIV risk.

## EDUCATION AND THE HIV EPIDEMIC

In examining the role of education in the HIV epidemic, there are a number of paradoxes. The first of these is that sub-Saharan African countries, which made the most progress in extending mass education to young women, are also among the top 15 countries most affected by the HIV epidemic, including Kenya, Namibia, South Africa, Zambia, and Zimbabwe. This paradox is expressed in Simon Gregson and his colleagues calling HIV/AIDS a "disease of development." It is Africa's *richest* but also most economically unequal countries such as South Africa and Botswana that have been particularly ravaged by HIV.[1]

Previous research on the links between educational attainment and HIV status has been largely statistical and mixed. Initially, the summary of studies by Judith Glynn and her colleagues on this paradox showed mixed results with some studies finding no statistical association and others finding positive associations between educational attainment and HIV status.[2] Jane Fortson, studying a number of surveys across Africa, found that education for all but the most elite is positively and significantly associated with higher HIV rates.[3] Other analyses suggest that the association between HIV and education varied according to the *length* of the epidemic in the country in question. The early stages of the epidemic showed positive associations, with more-educated people being more at risk of HIV. As the epidemic progresses, however, they argue that the relationship will be or is reversing to a negative association, with more-educated people better able to take advantage of new knowledge and change their behavior. While the evidence for this is still weak in most settings, the current consensus seems to support a coming reversal.[4] Two studies illustrate what appears to be a forthcoming trend. In Damien de Walque et al's study conducted in Uganda, the association between postprimary educational attainment and lower HIV risk became significant among young women in the eleventh annual survey round. Audrey Pettifor and her colleagues in a study in South Africa found that young women who began and then dropped out of high school had twice the HIV rates of those who completed high school. In this setting, young women who completed high school also had lower HIV rates compared to those who dropped out. However, in Kenya as a whole, women with no formal education have the lowest rates of HIV.[5]

The uncertain nature of the relationship between HIV and education is in some ways strange. We expect education to have an impact on HIV rates because of the almost common-sense understanding that education yields a multitude of health benefits including longer life expectancy and lower outcomes of many diseases, compared to those less educated—not just in developed countries, but also in developing countries. Further, there has, for some time now, been clear evidence that education has an effect on sexual behavior. Many demographers have shown the links between mass education and declines in fertility in the developing world, particularly among women with a high school education.[6] Changes in preferences regarding the number of children to have, as well as the increased use of Western contraceptives as a means to enact these preferences, are illustrations of the changed thinking, practice, and agency of educated women. Thus, the thinking goes, if education has such dramatic effects on one sexually transmitted condition—fertility—why not on HIV/AIDS?

Faith in schooling to come to the rescue in conquering social ills is not, on the face of it, misplaced when considering HIV.[7] School, the context in which mass education occurs, seems ideally suited to provide young women with greater access to life-saving education about HIV/AIDS compared to those women not in school. Indeed, one of the greatest successes of HIV campaigns in Africa is in education about HIV. As noted in chapter 4, over 90% of youth knew what HIV was and how to avoid getting it. In all the schools I visited, HIV/AIDS was a topic on the curriculum, and most students would have been exposed to many messages about HIV/AIDS throughout their educational career. A guidance-and-counseling teacher was often assigned to the task of educating youth about HIV/AIDS, and it was continually brought up as a topic in other classes, given the widespread effects the epidemic has had on Nyanza and Kenyan society. Indeed, given the way death shaped everyday life in Nyanza (discussed in chapter 3), including the attendant experience of having gone to funerals of relatives and friends who had died of HIV and the numerous students orphaned from HIV, "AIDS awareness" in this setting was something of a misnomer. School has clearly succeeded in the transmission of knowledge.

The paradox of educated women's high HIV rates in the face of widespread knowledge about HIV forces us to examine our assumptions about how we think education is supposed to impact young women and, ultimately, their HIV outcomes.[8] Rather than the predominant focus on school as a transmitter of HIV knowledge, of which it was highly successful, perhaps there are other ways to conceptualize school and what school does. School is not only a structural context in which formal education occurs; it is also charged by parents and communities with other tasks. Many parents, for example, liked boarding school for its ability to regulate their children's sexual behavior by monitoring students' movement and time use, and setting up rules, routines, and sanctions that, ideally, made it a logistical nightmare to set up rendezvous with sexual partners. This might suggest why Luo-Nyanza girls who made it through high school without dropping out had lower HIV rates compared to those who dropped out of high school and those who proceeded to college, who were well away from home and enjoying sexual freedom.[9] Additionally, school would ideally provide a supportive, normative environment reinforcing schoolgirls' choices to remain abstinent and postpone relationships until the completion of school because of the incompatibility seen between school and marriage, as well as motherhood. However, as I will illustrate in this chapter, structural processes and norms in school worked in gendered ways to produce just the opposite effect. I first turn to describing the pursuit of education in Kenya before examining in-school dynamics.

## THE PURSUIT OF EDUCATION

### The Rise of Mass Education

Mass modern education is a fairly recent development in many African societies. It is only in the 1980s and 1990s that mass primary education (defined by the percentage of children aged 15–19 who have completed over four years of schooling) reached 75% in a handful of African countries, including Botswana, Ghana, Kenya, South Africa, Cameroon, Tanzania, Zambia, and Zimbabwe. In the case of Kenya, Tanzania, and Zimbabwe, by 2000, gender gaps in enrollment had been almost completely eliminated, and mass schooling had been achieved in both urban and rural areas.[10] The impetus for this achievement in Kenya was the hope and faith placed by its people in education as a vehicle for modernization, development, and social mobility.[11] Some have argued that developing countries also had an interest in sparking such "enormous popular demand for schooling" as a way of gaining legitimacy.[12] Investment in schooling, particularly in the transition from the colonial to postcolonial era, and cultural changes occurring in the wake of this transition illustrated that "mass schooling has become a key strategy for signaling modern institutional change, particularly the coming of Western ideals and the arrival of mass opportunity. . . . By relying on signals of mass opportunity and meritocratic rules of getting ahead, the state can display Western ideals without directly attacking pre-modern economic interests and social organization."[13]

Education became increasingly important as colonial British civil servants left the country, leaving behind open positions for the few Kenyans who were educated to take their place. Thus, limited educational opportunities among Africans during the colonial period served to fuel demand for education once Kenya gained independence in 1963, and several jobs for the educated few opened up, as briefly discussed in chapter 3.[14]

The government response to Kenyans' thirst for education was reflected in the fact that by 1985, expenditures for education represented 35% of the country's budget. However, this was still not enough because of rapid population growth.[15] Kenya had one of the highest fertility rates in the world in 1978, with an average of almost eight children per woman.[16] Nyanza was not far from the national average, with seven children per woman.[17] These birth rates resulted in a large youth population in need of education. Indeed, in the face of the government's inability to cope with the fast-rising demand for not just primary but secondary education, Kenya's first and second presidents, Jomo Kenyatta and Daniel Arap Moi, encouraged communities to engage in self-help efforts to pool financial and labor resources and build their own schools. Women and women's groups, especially in rural areas, were a critical part of these so-called *harambee* school grassroots efforts; while women had limited access to leadership in these efforts, one estimate suggests that they formed 80% of the participants at fundraising events.[18] By 1987, out of a total of 2485 secondary schools in Kenya, 1497 (60%) were *harambee* schools,[19] a heavy investment by Kenyans in the education of their own children. The rapid rise in government and *harambee* schools was matched by a rapid increase in the private education industry. These investments as well as other private investments in higher-education institutions made Kenya's relatively extensive educational infrastructure attractive to students from many other African countries. By the end of the twentieth century, education in Kenya was a big foreign-exchange earner, with foreign students contributing Kshs 1 billion (about US $12.8 million).[20]

Despite the *harambee* wave, however, educational infrastructure development still did not keep pace with population growth.[21] Many students who graduated primary school were not able to gain access to secondary school simply because of a lack of space, as I discuss later. Further, structural-adjustment policies in Kenya, along with other African countries in the late 1980s, led to a decrease in public spending (including education) and a shift toward cost-sharing, which involved user fees.[22] In a context of economic recession and rising inequality, this resulted in the reduced ability of poor parents to afford fees and other educational expenses for their many children.[23]

## The Contemporary Pursuit of Education

Education continued to be valued in Kenya in the 1990s and early 2000s despite the challenges of school fees and a limited number of places in school. Between 1995 and 2006, over 90% of Kenyan children began primary school. (In Kenya, there are now eight years of primary school, culminating in the Kenya Certificate of Primary Education exam. This is followed by four years of secondary school [Form 1–Form 4], culminating in the Kenya Certificate of Secondary Education exam.) However, the transition rates from primary to secondary school remained at 50%, and many others dropped out before completion of secondary school. For those who managed to complete secondary education, entry into university was even more competitive. In 2000, only 5% of those who sat for the final high school exams got university places.[24]

To deal with the limitation of school fees, key election pledges subsequently implemented by the Kenyan government ahead of the elections in 2002 and 2007 were free primary education (in 2002) and free day and subsidized boarding secondary school education (in 2007). These policy shifts resulted in surprising trends; researchers found no net increase in enrollment in government primary schools between 1997 and 2006. Rather, a curious displacement was occurring. The policy clearly broadened access to education among the poor, with poorer students entering public schools. However, more affluent students were moving out of public and into private schools, which experienced rapid growth in both infrastructure and enrollment in both urban and rural areas.[25] The statistics from the latest KDHS survey (from 2010), which captured the beginning effects of the secondary-school fee burden reduction in 2007, suggests that, despite this relief, large-scale attrition from school has continued.

In the survey, among Kenyan youth (15–24 years old) as a whole, 6% of women and 2% of the men had no formal education. In contrast, every Luo-Nyanza youth (100%), regardless of gender, reported some formal education.[26] However, while higher proportions of Luo-Nyanza youth began school compared to the rest of the country, more of them, and women in particular, were delayed or stalled in their pursuit of education, with widening gaps at higher levels of education. While among Kenyan youth 58% of men and 64% of women had no more than a primary education, among Luo-Nyanza youth, slightly more men (62%) and women (70%) were at that level.[27] Fewer Luo-Nyanza women (8%) and men (10%) completed high school compared to women (13%) and men (17%) in the rest of Kenya.[28] Very few Kenyans made it to higher education institutions. By age 24, 2% and 4% of Luo-Nyanza women and men, respectively, and 5% and 6% of Kenyan women and men, respectively, reported higher education.[29] It is of note that, while there are still important gaps, significant progress in achieving gender parity in educational attainment in Kenya has been made.[30] Overall, however, these higher-education statistics suggest little change in the proportion of Kenyans going to university over the past decade, despite the expansion of the higher-educational system. Indeed, the statistics make it clear that Kenyans in high school are at the leading edge of a process of attrition throughout the educational process. In this next section, I explore in greater depth two of the major drivers of this large-scale attrition among the Luo of Nyanza despite their initial enthusiasm for school and the government fee payment and subsidies in 2007. The first is the continued expense of secondary schooling, particularly expenses related to school that are not part of tuition, and the second is the increasing disillusionment about the material returns of education.

*Expense of Schooling*

Many Luo parents were willing to go to great lengths to educate their children; however, putting children through school involved significant costs, especially relative to the increasingly difficult economic situation of average families. In the 1980s, the *"goro goro* economy" or "shilling economy" began to take hold in Nyanza when these high school youth were beginning elementary school. These phrases reflected the fact that the container *(goro goro)* used when buying products such as fish or corn to make the staple food grew smaller while the price remained the same.[31] Further economic shocks occurred in the 1990s when a number of industries including the breweries, the railroad, and British American Tobacco shut down or mechanized their systems, resulting in mass layoffs of workers. The government and many parastatals including the Ministry of Works also laid off people as they tried to reduce the size of the labor force and increase efficiency as well as cut the ministry budget as part of the "economic restructuring" mandated by structural adjustment.[32] As noted in chapter 1, while Kenya's GDP per capita was about $1000 a year,[33] District Development Plans in the Nyanza districts where I conducted my research estimated that 53%–69% of their populations lived on less than $1 a day. While some parents in urban areas had salaried jobs, many had small businesses that brought in highly variable income; in rural areas, many parents and guardians were peasant farmers. The situation seemed well summed up by one student who simply said, "you find most of the parents are not able."

While the burden of school fees has been reduced or almost completely removed now, the statistics cited earlier—showing that over 80% of Kenyans do not complete high school—suggest that large-scale attrition up to and throughout high school has continued. As noted earlier, school infrastructure did not expand fast enough to absorb primary-school graduates looking to enroll in secondary schools, which were now free. There was no increase in the number of schools by 2006, and there was also a decline in the number of teachers. Thus, the teacher-student ratio in government schools increased as crowding in schools became the norm.[34] This new reality has meant that, despite the fee relief for government schools, there is increased competition for few places. Parents whose children do not get a place in a government secondary school have to pay school fees to get their children into the expanding number of private schools, where the net increase in enrollment has occurred. Private schools are also perceived to be of better quality and are important for parents who are hoping to give their children the best chance of getting into university, where the competition is even more fierce. Additionally, while students going to government day secondary schools did not pay school fees, those going to boarding schools only received partial tuition fee reductions. Boarding schools were also perceived to be better and less distracting for students than day schools and were the preferred option for many parents. Thus, even in this new reality, for aspirational parents, who are likely to live in the wealthier households more affected by HIV, school fees continue to be an important part of the family budget. In this situation, while the reality of 2006 I describe in the next section has changed somewhat for some, for many others the challenges faced by students and parents contending with school fees during fieldwork continue to be relevant today, not just in Kenya, but in many other African countries where no such government secondary-school fee subsidies exist.

School fees at the randomly selected high schools I visited ranged from Kshs 13,600 ($194 a year) in the day school to Kshs 24,000 ($340 a year) in the boarding schools,[35] and the average Nyanza family, as noted earlier, had about seven children. A little education for every child might have been seen as a better strategy than longer education for a few, and the decision regarding which child to pull out of school when was often gendered. However, even for the few, with poverty levels so high in this province, and some tuition requiring a substantial proportion of their income, it is not surprising that many parents defaulted on the fees.[36] To give an illustration of this, in one of the schools, the "fee problem" was posted outside the principal's office for all to see. (See table 1.)

Fees at the school were Kshs 22,900 ($327) for boarders and Kshs 13,600 ($194) for day students. As the table illustrates, students owed the school almost half a million Kenya shillings ($5994), a large amount of money for a rural school to be operating without. While the government was responsible for paying teachers' salaries and gave subsidies to schools,[37] operating expenses were often generated through the school fee system. Considering this school had about 200 students, this means that almost 40% of the students had the "fee problem." This represented a typi-

*Table 1*    "Serious Fee Payment" in a Boarding Secondary School in
             Rural Nyanza

| 18 students | Form 4 | Owed a total of | 83,625 | $1194 |
|---|---|---|---|---|
| 19 students | Form 3 | Owed a total of | 141,600 | $2023 |
| 16 students | Form 2 | Owed a total of | 81,800 | $1169 |
| 22 students | Form 1 | Owed a total of | 112,575 | $1608 |
| 75 students | | Owing a grand total of | 419,600 | $5994 |

cal example of the situation faced by almost all of the schools I visited. The
Kenyan government had set up a bursary system to give merit- and need-
based assistance to students. In addition, many secondary schools were
kept afloat by money paid by nongovernmental organizations such as Care
and World Vision in support of a fraction of the over 300,000 orphans in
the province (see chapter 3). In some schools, almost half the students
were single or double orphans. These organizations were often a school's
most reliable fee payers.[38] Orphans were particularly vulnerable to attrition from school, not just because of their dependence on relatives or a
single parent for school fees, but also because the demand for their labor
at home was high. Girls in particular could be pulled from home to engage
in domestic work or care for a sick parent.[39] Thus, the provision of school
fees and other support to the host family from these organizations and
other donors could often mean the difference between an orphan girl staying home and doing housework, or continuing on with her education.

In most schools, being sent home at one point or another for school fees
was a common experience. Parents may be able to come up with partial
fees, allowing the student to start school, but the parent would then be
unable to come up with the rest in time, and so the student was sent home
until the balance could be paid. In this manner, an education characterized
by many interruptions resulting in months or years of delay was the norm.
It was not unusual to find youth in their mid- to late teens in primary
school or those in their early 20s in high school.[40] The sight of students
leaving school at odd times of day and year was common, and they were a
frequent topic of conversation among passengers on public transportation
vehicles when they observed students entering the bus, or *matatu*. Student
absences were sometimes strictly enforced by the schools, as a high school

girl, Christine, described: "I was lacking in money to pay [for] school. So most of the time I was spending at home and sometimes you can try just to steal a day in school and if you're gotten there, you'll be beaten."[41]

While students were home, the scramble to find fees was a family production. A community member explained, "parents just struggle to get the school fees and the children also get involved in activities like fetching firewood and taking to markets to sell and boys can burn charcoal and sell to get money." Other parents would contact relatives in other parts of Kenya or outside of the country for assistance. The following excerpt from an interview with a high school boy, Bramson, illustrates the typical educational journey for students in this setting:

> My dad was . . . being held up [in jail]. My mum, she could not raise the money for my education. . . . So I spent two years at home because of lack of fees. My uncle could not kind of raise that money. And by then, my aunt who is in [the] States I could not get to contact her. So we just went like that until my dad was released the following year. So we tried looking for a school [and] we found one but then the money was not available because my dad had still not settled down. So that second year also passed. So third year, my aunt sent for him some cash and I was fortunate to get admitted in some school. . . . So I learnt there for Form 1, then again, fees problem cropped up, I dropped, and the whole of second term I wasn't in school. So I was forced to go back during third term and they declined to take me in unless I repeat Form 1.

The family proceeded to look for a school that would let him continue on to Form 2. While his situation, with a father in jail, was unusual, the struggle to find fees, relying on extended family to contribute, and the years of interrupted education were not.

It was also clear during fieldwork that there were many costs beyond school fees that parents had to incur. Table 2 provides a summary of several other annual expenses common to all the schools that emerged in interviews. As the table indicates, in addition to school fees, going to school also generated a multitude of needs. Parents were expected to pay for school uniforms and students were not allowed to attend school without it. Indeed, David Evans and colleagues found that in a fee-free environment, primary school students' absteentism from school reduced by almost half when they were given school uniforms (as part of a randomized trial). The reductions were even higher for students who had not

*Table 2*   Annual High School Expenses per Child in a Sample of
Secondary Schools in Nyanza Province, Kenya

| Item | Kenya Shillings | US Dollars |
| --- | --- | --- |
| School fees | 13,000–24,000 | $200–340 |
| School uniforms | 1000+ | $14+ |
| "Shopping" | 3000–6000 | $43–86 |
| Lunch for day school | 2700 (10/day) | $40 |
| Textbooks | 3000 | $43 |
| TOTAL | 22,700–36,700 | $324–$524 |

previously had a uniform. Esther Duflo and colleagues also found that girls given free uniforms were less likely to drop out of school. Both of these studies, combined with findings in this setting, suggest that it was a significant barrier to going to school.[42] In this setting, a uniform set would include a skirt or trousers, a shirt, a tie, a sweater and/or blazer, a pair of socks, and a particular kind of leather shoe chosen by the school; sometimes a sports uniform was also included, which was a skirt or shorts and a shirt. In a particularly poignant moment for me at the beginning of the school year, I was sitting in a principal's foyer waiting for an interview at one school. The office was crowded with parents, guardians, and prospective students who were being handed out uniforms after the parents had paid. Students would then go and change into them. One female prospective student was struggling to put on her tie, and I offered to help. As I fixed the tie, my mind took me back to my own school days, as I remembered the excitement of putting on a school uniform, and getting used to these strange new clothes, representing my new status as a schoolgirl.

Shopping, especially for boarding school students, would include toiletries and laundry materials (for example, toothpaste, toothbrush, and laundry detergent to hand wash clothes), clothing other than the uniform, food items (if these were allowed in school), and so on. In many schools, students also had to buy their own textbooks and exercise books for taking notes in class. Thus, total costs for putting one student through high school could reach as high as $520 in a given year (and almost $200 without school fees included)—a significant financial investment, given the average household income and family size. In addition, many schools also charged ad hoc mandatory fees throughout the school year including "teacher motivation" fees, building development fees, and so on to supplement teacher salaries (which were static because of government freezes), or to pursue various improvement projects in the school.

### Disillusionment with Returns on an Investment in Education

Unfortunately for many, the huge struggle to support a student through school was increasingly less likely to be matched by the well-paid white-collar employment aspired to by a high school graduate and their family. Indeed, there was a sense of widespread disillusionment with the returns of education, both in terms of stable jobs and in terms of higher income relative to the uneducated or lesser educated. This decline in returns was driven by structural-adjustment policies that resulted in a reduction in formal-sector jobs, as well as by demography, with increasing numbers of people competing for few jobs. The spread of mass primary and secondary education was coupled with an economy that was not expanding at a rate that could accommodate the graduates. This resulted in a rising number of the "educated unemployed."[43] Tracer studies conducted at the time showed a slowing down in absorption of school graduates into the labor force.[44] Further, qualification escalation and certificate devaluation began to occur, with higher education needed for lower-level jobs. Thus, unlike parents and grandparents, for whom even completion of half of high school would be sufficient for a civil servant job (see chapter 3), now perhaps a university degree was needed. Its impact on the availability of white-collar jobs led to a changing cost-benefit analysis when considering whether to keep children in school and a different valuation of the opportunity costs of children's labor. So children might be pulled out of school to help with farming and other economic activities or to help care for the family, especially if there were sick relatives or parents. As noted earlier, orphans were particularly vulnerable to being pulled out of school for these reasons.[45] I discuss the transition out of school and into the workforce in chapter 6.

Thus, education was seen less and less as an effective means toward salaried employment and financial independence, and there was a clear generational difference in the experience of education. The climate for the classes of the generations of the 1990s and 2000s was in some ways starkly different from their parents and grandparents who grew up during the colonial and early postcolonial era, who recalled the educated having their pick of jobs, and who perceived clear differences between the educated and the uneducated. In Luo-Nyanza, even while many parents were making great sacrifices to educate their children, and while their strong belief in education persisted, a thread of ambivalence colored their comments. Many saw their sons and daughters return home after high school to sit in idleness without jobs for extended periods of time, leading them to feel that the link between education and good jobs and a steady source of income over the decades had become tenuous. As a man in his 80s noted in frustration and sadness, "Education is expensive. After that expensive education, there are no jobs. So the children who are educated have lost their way and they get into different things. We have a problem because they are back with us in the house. They come to disturb us parents. You had educated her or him, you have no money."[46] Another noted, *"pok amadho chach somo"* (I have not yet drunk the tea of education). In other words, he was still waiting to see the payoff from education.

It is in this context of a tension between the expected material returns of education and increasing disillusionment about the potential of reaching it that I will describe how gendered life-and-death outcomes for young people resulted. First, I show how school through gendered processes *produced* consuming women and, thus, women with increased incentive to engage in transactional relationships. Next, I show how the context of school inadvertently *facilitated* transactional relationships with older partners. Finally, I discuss the dueling normative systems young women were engaging with and having to choose between as they navigated the school environment in pursuit of their education.

## SCHOOL AND THE PRODUCTION OF CONSUMING WOMEN
### The Language of "Needs" and the Construction of Gendered Needs

Throughout chapter 4, when young people were talking about the centrality of money in relationships for sex, they often referred to "needs." For example, needs were mentioned in reference to quarrels arising in a sexual relationship when a boyfriend did not provide: "if he fails to *satisfy your needs*. Maybe you wanted even let's say 200 shillings [$2.85] to *satisfy your needs*. Then here comes a case where he may even tell you that I don't have that [right] now. And then maybe you know that he has the money. Then he is just refusing to give it to you. Then that might end up with quarrels." Needs were mentioned in explaining why girls might engage in transactional relationships: "sometimes your parents cannot afford some money to buy for us *things girls need*. So you can go and have sex with a boy so he can give you money to buy your things." Young men would also complain about the needs of girls, as one noted: "I had a girlfriend. She was very expensive in that she will *need always* sanitary towels [pads], oils that will make her comfortable, and some clothes that [I could not] afford, so having a girlfriend [was] just a problem and very expensive . . . she was [the kind of girl for whom] the relationship couldn't have continued if I couldn't provide." Another young man said: "We *need more* than girls because *everything that girls can need*, they get three-quarters from us."

Generally, when we think of "needs," especially in a context of poverty where most families live on less than a dollar a day, it is certainly plausible to think about girls' needs as food on the table and to more easily classify their relationships with providing men as "survival sex." However, for most of my respondents who were going to or had passed through school, their families were at least able to provide food, shelter, clothing, and other "survival" provision. Thus, these were not survival "needs"; they were merely constructed as such. They were, rather, needs for consumption goods above and beyond basics. Indeed, "the ideology of consumerism entail[s] the creation and promotion of "false needs," that is, the fostering of the need for things not strictly necessary for survival."[47]

What was also striking, and underscored this *social* construction of needs, was the gendered nature of what were considered needs. Indeed, it was "common sense" that girls needed more than boys. For example, a schoolgirl, Jatella, noted: "Boys don't have so much needs like girls. . . . You find that . . . when schools open, you see girls carrying very big boxes and the boys, just one bag." Similarly, a schoolboy, Goma, noted in reference to girls, "I think their apparatus is big. They need a lot of things so that they can be satisfied. A girl cannot be satisfied the way she is. But when she applies some things [like skin lotion] that is when she will be satisfied."

The high school boy was not only highlighting girls' greater needs for things, but also suggesting that not having these needs met would lead to a certain discontent and hunger in girls. Indeed, boys often contrasted girls' need for *immediate* satisfaction with their own ability to *postpone* their desires for things with phrases such as "boys can survive," "we can do without," and "girls want things easy, while boys are more ready to kind of sacrifice." Boys were essentially "doing gender" in constructing a masculinity of restraint in the face of consumer desire (which was somewhat convenient, since they were broke). A list of boys' perceived needs included soap, laundry detergent, toothbrush and toothpaste, and a little pocket money. When pressed, some went beyond this to note larger purchases, but even these were constructed as "basic needs." For example, Johnson noted, "A person may want to have what a friend has, like a radio cassette, bicycle, though a bicycle can help you get basic needs. And another basic need is hospital, if you can get money to go to hospital when you are sick." Another young man, Jeremiah, noted, "a person should be able to eat. You must be able to dress well so that even if you are among your peers you don't get ashamed, and a place to sleep and proper beddings."

That the importance of dressing well was noted as a need not only belied the "basic" nature of boys' needs, but also reflected a type of "uniform" that the elders they were looking up to seemed to conform to. As I walked through Luo towns and villages throughout fieldwork, the standard dress for a Luo man of a certain age, regardless of wealth, invariably included a suit jacket, a hat, and a cane, even if his trousers might be tattered, his shoes torn, and his shirt worn.

Girls' lists would often be much longer and more elaborate, including items such as cosmetics, skin lotion, face powder, and new shoes. An illustrative example is shown in the following excerpt from a focus group interview with girls at a boarding school whom I asked to list some of these needs, after they said that they had many. After listing the same "basics" as the boys, the conversation continued:

AGNES: And don't forget the cosmetics.
MAGGIE: Yeah.

SANYU:    Cosmetics? And that's a need? *[Laughter.]*

AGNES:    I think so. In a girls school like this, for example, you're not even bought for such things like Fair [Fair and Lovely is a popular face cream], [or] powder, and you come and you find, for example, Mary, she has all those things but me I don't have. You know she looks somehow—

MAGGIE:   Beautiful.

AGNES:    Beautiful. You might say you, you also want.

ROSIE:    Yeah.

SANYU:    So won't she share with you? Can't you ask her, "Hey, could I have some?"

AGNES:    Every day? *[Laughter.]*

JENNY:    *Atakutia mudomoni.* [She will pout her lips at you.] *[Laughter.]*

In another interview, a schoolgirl, Anita, noted, "Girls need a lot of things because a girl will want to dress properly, she will want to bathe well, and use good oil, she will want to have proper shoes, and to be fashionable and trendy, she will want to plait her hair, and the rest that you think that a girl can use. So I think that girls need more than boys." Two young men, James and Ben, in another context reflected the same difference. James observed, "You know boys, they can even have three clothes, but a girl can't sit with just three clothes." Ben added, "[Girls] love money because they can't ask their parents but they like these small small things like makeup, their needs are high. So they love money to buy these small things."

There was no disagreement between the genders about who "needed" more, even though boys also had consumer desires, like "dress[ing] properly." In other words, despite boys and girls *both* being drawn into the culture of consumption, the discursive language around who was most entangled in it—indeed, entangled to the point of "need"—was clearly gendered and considered part of the very nature of girls.

### School Structure and Gendered Needs

The construction of gendered needs was enhanced by the social structure of school. It was an institution that brought large numbers of girls, often from a wide range of social backgrounds and family structures, together in one space, either daily or in the same residence for boarding schools. As illustrated in the excerpts earlier, school was where "new needs" were discovered, and girls could and did compare among themselves the extent to which perceived needs that seemed to be collectively shared were met. It was one thing to share a product with another girl one time, but such sharing could not continue forever, especially if the product could run out. Peer groups, key microstructures within schools, provided key venues for this to occur,[48] since they could contribute to young women's dissatisfaction with what they had and create a longing to have what others had. As Sarah put it, "when you see other girls, the way they put on, [you think,] 'what about me?'" This sentiment could lead girls into relationships so that they could get money to look like others. Granita said, for example, "Girls like admiring, so you may find a girl walking around the street and looking at fellow girls who have things that she doesn't have, so you may find that since the girl doesn't have money, it will force her to play sex with a boy, so she will just play that sex to get money to buy things she saw."

School also made differences between groups apparent. A girl who was out of school would only notice that she lacked something when she went into town or if a girl in her village acquired something that the first girl liked. In a school setting, however, differences between girls were regularly made evident, especially if this difference was something worn every day. For one schoolgirl, being teased because she was wearing homemade shoes instead of the store-bought shoes that were in fashion that year was a painful and humiliating experience. When she went home that holiday, new shoes had become a need. Similarly, not having money to buy a small meal with her friends meant that a schoolgirl would feel excluded, and money to go on such outings would become a need. Allison Pugh discusses how young people's consumption desires are not just about wanting to possess material things; they are also a way of participating in their school culture and attaining social visibility among their peers. By having what others also have, they are able not only to participate in discussions about shared experiences, but also, more powerfully, to feel like they socially belong or are fully social citizens in their environments and not excluded. She shows how parents' recognition of the meaning behind children's consumption desires compels them to purchase products and experiences for their children that they may not otherwise want to.[49] In this setting, peer influence was a critical factor, particularly in a school setting, since groups of girls could share their experiences with one another and create normative environments for transactional sex relationships to meet what they all considered necessities, as I discuss later.

## The Nature of "Needs"

In many of the statements quoted, not only was the variety of girls' needs highlighted, but also their frequency and volume. Not just one nice piece of clothing was needed, but several. Plaited hair would only stay looking good for a short period of time before it would have to be taken out and redone or have a new hairstyle put in. After bathing, young women liked to oil their skin with Vaseline so their skin would shine; however, it came in a container that would soon need replenishing. These were not one-off needs, but rather *continual* needs, all of which required continual *funding*. Several older women noted that there was an increase in the volume of things young women said they needed. Amollo, for example, said that when she was young, many girls had only one dress, and when they were traveling, they would borrow a second dress from the neighbor. This was a period when shifts were being made toward modern types of clothing; thus, women of their time were only just starting to acquire them.[50] To them and many others, the needs of young women today were seen to have dramatically increased. In contrast, beyond the "basics" like toothpaste and soap, many of boys' needs were one-time and durable items like a radio-cassette player or a bicycle. Hence, a one-time gift to a boy would result in long-term satisfaction, whereas a one-time gift to a girl would only be good until her desired product was finished, and she would need to be "satisfied" again.

Adjudicating among stated needs to determine "true" and "false" needs becomes complicated when considering the most consistently mentioned need among girls in school—sanitary pads.[51] Are they a need or a want? The answer to this question differed by generation in ways that were consequential for school-going women. While the price ranged from Kshs 45 to 80 ($.64–$1.14) per packet of eight, this was not always considered a "need" worth including in school "shopping" by parents, guardians, and donors. Sanitary pads (along with other toiletries like deodorant and toothpaste) are a classic example of a "modern" product that cannot be washed, reused, or in any way recycled. Once the product acquires the status of "need" in a girl's mind, she becomes tied to a product that generates recurring monthly expenses for her entire reproductive life and, consequently, a recurring monthly need for money to purchase it.

For centuries, Luo women have had alternative solutions for menstruation that worked for them, even with fairly active lives trading, doing vigorous agricultural work, walking many miles, and so on, and many women in the community would use rags and other traditional solutions. However, among many young women, especially those who were school going or had been exposed to school, sanitary pads were considered a need. Gracia, a day scholar, used to save up money given to her for public transport and chose instead to walk a long distance to school to save up for sanitary pads, which her guardian did not provide for her. A schoolgirl wholly dependent on parents or guardians who were already making great sacrifices to pay for her high school tuition and associated fees would have to rely on pocket money, if given it, or find alternative sources of money if she did not get sanitary pads in her shopping.

While from a Westernized, "modern" perspective one might more easily sympathize with Luo schoolgirls seeing sanitary pads as a "need," the point I want to emphasize is that products as needs can be arbitrarily designated: sanitary pads had become necessities for schoolgirls and were new "needs." However, once they had become a "need" in a girl's mind, not having the product would create acute discontent in a young woman's mind and motivate action to satisfy that need. Thus, a teenage schoolgirl, Maria, said, "if the family is poor, you know as girls we *need* several things, but if the family can't provide all this, the girl will be *forced* to search for them somewhere else" (my emphasis). The stated compulsion to search for money noted by this and many other schoolgirls matched their sense that the things desired were "needs" as opposed to "wants." Regardless of whether these were really "needs," the fact that young women *perceived* them as needs was consequential for both their pursuit and their justification of the means they engaged in to enable consumption and consumer satisfaction.

## EDUCATION AND MODERNITY

School is presumed to fulfill a number of different roles, including cultural transmission, socialization (behavioral, moral, and cultural), and social selection.[52] And these features are not lost on citizens in developing countries who fully recognize that schools are engaged in taking "traditional" youth and transforming them into "modern" adults. School uniforms are visible markers of this process in motion—hence the pride felt when first wearing one. School does not only teach skills such as English literacy in order to enable citizens to engage in modern and global economies; it also inculcates in participants different sets of habits and lifestyles compared to those who do not go.[53] Bruce Fuller, for example, describes a girl in a boarding school in Zambia who had to wear pajamas to bed, use cutlery, and eat a very different diet, noting, "While Chimtali obviously enjoyed becoming modern, she had not suspected that secondary school would require such deep changes in daily habits."[54] Moving from rags to sanitary pads is certainly a deep and perhaps irreversible or hard-to-give-up change in monthly habits.

School was an institution charged with the production of modern subjects.[55] Further, going to school was not just about becoming modern women, but also about demonstrating this transformation through engaging in *practices* that marked their difference. Village girls could use rags during menstruation; schoolgirls wore sanitary pads. Village girls could make their own oil for their skin and face, and their own soap using ingredients gathered from the natural environment; schoolgirls bought Vaseline Intensive Care Lotion, Fair and Lovely face cream, and Imperial Leather soap. Village girls were comfortable in their natural beauty, with dark skin, long necks, and teeth with a gap *(singare)*; schoolgirls wore makeup. Engaging in these practices, however, carried a dilemma: a schoolgirl was a girl who consumed, and consumption required money that, in many cases, she had less access to compared with boys, as I will show in the next chapter. In the process of transforming "traditional girls" into "modern schoolgirls," school also, inadvertently, produced consuming women. Consuming young women had desires that could only be satisfied by consumption, desires that were considered necessities and integral to schoolgirls' transformation. The project of modernity, the implicit work of school, then, was arguably bound up with consumption—consumption that many could not afford.

For young women, transactional relationships emerged as part of their toolkit of strategies[56] to gain access to money. Even while relationships often involved love and trust (as described in the previous chapter), the centrality of money to the project of modernity also supported a logic of partner change in the absence of provision, and indeed a preference for the partners who were most capable of provision. This makes sense of Sacha's comment in chapter 1 that "if you find somebody who cannot provide all these *necessities* . . . the girl may switch to the next man she thinks might provide it. So that's the reason as to why the girls move from one man to another, and get infected to this disease easier" (my emphasis).

## FACILITATING TRANSACTIONAL RELATIONSHIPS

There were other ways in which school complicated young women's safe transition through school. In reflecting on young women's HIV risk in a focus group among young women going to vocational postsecondary school, Leila noted: "I think education can also be a cause, especially on the side of the ladies. Because you find nowadays, ladies don't agree to get married before they finish their education *and in the process of being educated*, they will get into sexual activities which can make them to get the disease" (my emphasis). When young women thought about connections between school and HIV, it was less about the role of school in helping them learn about HIV or about the content of their education, and more about the complicated process of becoming educated. In the following section, I unpack this process showing how school strategies to prevent girls from sexual relationships often backfired in unanticipated ways.

Toward the end of an interview with a schoolgirl, May, who had lost both parents, I asked her:

SANYU: Is there anything in the main discussion that you think I didn't cover that you think is important? Like issues of education and issues of employment and issues of HIV?

MAY: Not really but you find that, let's say, a girl, an orphan, the family she comes from does not support her, her education. Then she happens to find a man who is working, then this man maybe decides to, I don't know, tries to joke around with her life, maybe pretending to be taking care of, will be taking care of her, maybe taking her back to school. Then you find that this working man impregnates the girl, then dumps her there. Now you see the parents, the family from where you come from, they'll assume that it's through your immoral behaviors that you got [became] a victim, but maybe it was not your wish. Maybe it was lack of support, lack of money to get your basic needs. So I don't know how that one can be helped, and quite a number have [become] victims as a result of that.

SANYU:  So do you know, like, personal examples?

MAY:  Yeah, I had a friend of mine. Her parents passed away and she was only one in the family. Then she had to go, she comes from around [here]. She had to go and stay with an aunt who also comes from around here. Then the aunt was just less concerned about her, not providing anything, you're just seeing her there. Then she happened to [become] a victim of a certain man who was working. Then the man promised the girl to take her back to school, she was in Form 2. Then I don't know what happened, but the man dumped her after impregnating the girl. Now she had to give birth. Then the family complained that she is being immoral, something like that. But she is not going to school nowadays. She is just staying there, with her child there.

In May's narrative, we see how the working man began a relationship with her friend Rachel by promising to support her education, thus demonstrating his care and concern for her.[57] Once Rachel got pregnant, however, she was abandoned by the man and had to leave school, and was now at home with her child. For this former schoolgirl, she had already beaten the odds in Luo-Nyanza by being among the 30% with more than a primary-school education, but in the process of trying to become part of the 8% who complete high school, a relationship with a working man had *both* enabled and derailed her. Attrition from school in her case was due both to a lack of fees that resulted in the interruption from school and a period at home, and to a subsequent vulnerability to the approach from the working man. By offering to pay school fees, the man was showing "concern" and helping with instrumental support lacking from her relatives.[58] The pregnancy and birth that ensued ended her pursuit of education altogether. This story also highlights the contradictions inherent in young women's higher education. Relationships with providing men enabled them to go further than their parents and guardians could afford in their education—hence the family silence or tacit support of supportive boyfriends.[59] But they also put these schoolgirls at risk for pregnancy in the short term (which often led to dropping out of school and, in this case, family condemnation), and HIV in the long term. The educational process was thus one in which the contradictions and ambivalence among parents and guardians around transactional relationships played out.


## REGULATING SCHOOLGIRL SEXUAL BEHAVIOR

In an effort to prevent girls from having sexual relationships, schools would often attempt to control girls' mobility in school, and in many cases they were successful. The danger came when girls left school. Girls in day school would sneak out of their home in the evenings to go to the clubs to meet men, as described in chapter 4. For girls in boarding school, however, there was an irony in their description of how the strict rules governing their mobility in school increased their motivation to rebel during school holidays. (The typical school year in Kenya begins in January and is characterized by three terms with a break for Easter, a month break in August, and two-month break between November and January. National Certificate exams are taken in November.) A girl in boarding school, Crispa, drolly said, "when we are in boarding school, we are prevented from a lot of things. [When] we are in places where we can go outside, we try to do all the things that we were missing. Things that are very risky."

A common joke contrasted students in all-girl boarding schools with those in mixed-gender or day schools, and noted that the girls in boarding school were the most likely to engage in sexual relationships outside of school because they had been deprived of boys. (The influx of mobile phones, however, had begun to undermine the teachers' confidence in their ability to prevent girls in boarding school from engaging in relationships in school. Personal phones, given to them by their male partners, were being used to set up meeting points and times with men outside of school. School watchmen could always be bribed.)

The structure of the school calendar played a role in shaping the timing of girls' relationships because of the challenge of conducting them in school. Schoolgirls would note their particular vulnerability in engaging in transactional relationships when the end of holidays was nearing and they were about to go back to school to rejoin their schoolmates. The long two-month holiday (from November to January) coincided with the mass exodus of city-based Luo men in Nairobi and Mombasa (two large Kenyan cities) back to Nyanza province to visit relatives for Christmas. The men, flush with cash that they were bringing home to families, would engage in relationships on the side, while young women would receive money for their back-to-school shopping. So normalized was this assumption of girls' sexual relationships over the long holidays that several schools institutionalized pregnancy tests when students returned at the beginning of the school year. One student wryly described how, in her school, the principal actually congratulated the students because no one was found to be pregnant that year.

The concern about girls' relationships with working men was often expressed in terms of relationships with men outside of school—in the clubs, local neighborhoods, and fish-landing beaches. However, many of the older men with money who were immediately available to young women were not *outside* of school in clubs and local neighborhoods, but teachers *within* the school.

## TEACHER-STUDENT RELATIONSHIPS

Lizzy, a high school student, described teacher-student relationships in her school and how they had personally affected her. During the interview, I asked her:

SANYU: And what about boys, do they have many relationships as well?

LIZZY: Yeah they do. And then you find that if a girl refuses a boy they start rumormongering about you. They say things which are not true. Like in this school we even have teachers who they try to get the students but if you refuse they start talking about you . . .

SANYU: So even teachers?

LIZZY: Yeah, in this school even teachers. And actually our principal is trying to control that. I can say that—

SANYU: He is aware also?

LIZZY: Yeah, he is aware and he is trying to control it seriously.

SANYU: How, how is he?

LIZZY:   He calls you, he talks to you, and then I think he calls the same teacher and talks to the same teacher.

SANYU:   And does that have repercussions on the students afterward?

LIZZY:   Yeah.

SANYU:   How?

LIZZY:   You know *[chuckles]*, actually these things happen. You will see that the student is there, but maybe she will be there but the mind is not there. Because if you know somebody, they say this about you, "The teacher wants you actually and you refuse!" Then the teacher starts talking about you. You will hate the teacher and obviously you will hate the subject.

The interview progressed to a discussion of other topics. At the end of the interview, I turned the tape off, preparing to leave. However, at that point, Lizzy began to share details about her current dilemma, and I realized that the situation she was alluding to in the interview was about her. She had been approached for a relationship by two different teachers on separate occasions when she arrived at the school—new girls, she said, were particularly vulnerable. She told both of them no. One accepted her decision and instead became a friendly and supportive teacher as she proceeded through school. The other, however, persisted in trying to convince her to have a relationship with him. Lizzy told the headmaster about the situation and he talked to the teacher in question, but in the end, he was not dismissed and carried on teaching in the school. Because the teacher taught mathematics, a subject she would have to pass in order to go to university, she was forced to go to crucial classes and regularly face a teacher who now resented her and tried to make life difficult for her. It did not help that through rumormongering, everyone knew about the situation. She was not sure what more to do, since she had already told the principal.

Jacinta, a girl in another high school, described the same problem: "Sometimes, like now, we're in a girls school and let's say a male teacher proposes for you to be the girlfriend and you refuse, you know most of the time he will be frustrating you in school and you will not be all that free even in your classes. Now what if Mr. so and so [is] teaching science and maths, you'll switch off completely. Yeah, you'll switch off." Many students felt that reporting the teacher would result in sanctions on them in terms of lower grades or being failed in the class. At a visit to one school, a female teacher noted how, in casual conversations in the faculty room, male teachers would note about some female students, "that one is ready for marriage," to laughter by all; but it was clear in her retelling of this anecdote that she saw this as a troubling trend in her school and that it greatly concerned her.

Given the qualitative nature of this study, it was difficult to establish just how widespread these relationships were. In one school, I tried to do this by asking a focus group how many girls in a group of ten would have had a relationship with a teacher. They said three. In other settings, it had become common sense. "Where male teachers are there, [you] can't miss [such relationships]." School sometimes created a normative environment supporting "grooving with the teachers."

The widespread nature of accounts of teacher-student relationships in work by Africanist researchers suggests that the prevalence of these relationships is not trivial.[60] Students described many of the teachers as married, and said that girls engaged in these relationships because of fear and because of the money that teachers gave as part of the relationship. Money was then used for school shopping and as additional pocket money to meet the needs that parents and family could not or would not. The amounts given ranged from Kshs 25 to Kshs 2000 ($0.35–$28.50) every term. They said that students in these relationships rarely if ever got pregnant, presumably because the teachers provided them with birth control, or if they did, the teacher would deny responsibility and it was blamed on men outside the school.

The challenge for teachers in rural schools in particular was the fact that in villages and communities where most parents were farmers and earned money itinerantly, the teachers were paid by the government and thus got money on a monthly basis. They were often the only salaried individuals in a community. The day of the month when teachers got paid was widely known in communities. Teachers in remote areas would often have to make a special visit to a town or the city to go to the bank to withdraw their pay. Long lines could be found outside ATMs in Kisumu, Nyanza's capital, on such days. Teachers' "ties of dependence" to their communities created obligations for them to share their relative wealth to maintain goodwill.[61] There were many ways in which teachers did this; some female teachers, for example, mentioned how they hired locals to work their farms and paid them money. In this light, some male teachers were seen to "help" local widows through transactional relationships, leaving the widow with financial support for her children. Students in turn benefited with financial assistance.

What makes teacher-student relationships particularly devastating now is HIV. Just one infected teacher having relationships with students could wreak havoc. One teacher, Alice, told me of a girl in standard six (Grade 6) infected by a male teacher, noting that primary school was worse in terms of the extent of teacher-student relationships. "In fact primary is worse . . . because you find even the teachers themselves are going with these girls. But because these girls are just too young, they don't know how to say no. 'Cause if you say no you'll be caned. They are giving in at class six."

In another instance, a high school boy, Chris, in a different district described a school-wide HIV test conducted in a neighboring provincial girls school.

> Recently the principal of that school decided to make the students undergo an HIV test. So they did that and when the results came, it came that more than a quarter of the school were HIV positive. The main reason most of them were infected was their teacher. There was a teacher there who was HIV positive, and the girls were yearning for academic excellence. So he would call the girls and say 'you come and visit me at one time.' . . . The teacher was teaching them but after that the teacher would bed them. So they ended up being infected.[62]

In an interview with an HIV-positive young woman, Kamimi, who was out of school, she revealed that when she was 16, she married a 30-year-old teacher because she did not have fees to continue school, and she said that the marriage was of her own volition. She was one of those girls, described in the previous chapter, who would "just go because the family cannot afford." She said, "Me I think it is my husband who gave [HIV] to me. He was having affairs with many girls." She said that she discovered he was having affairs after she had stayed with him for a while, and that he even brought some of the girls to their home. He himself admitted to her that he gave her the disease and told her not to worry, saying that many people had the disease and were surviving on antiretroviral drugs, which had begun to be rolled out in 2006. A student noted, "when teachers think they have the disease they cheat on girls."[63]

While male teachers have higher rates of HIV compared to those who are not teachers, this is not because teachers are necessarily high risk in and of themselves. Rather, their apparently higher HIV prevalence is a function more of their mobility, relative wealth, and age profile than of the fact that they teach specifically.[64] Teachers are generally wealthier, and most are in their 30s and 40s. The standard qualification for primary-school teachers in Kenya is a teaching-college education, while university qualifications are expected for secondary-school teachers. They are the largest workforce in Kenya, with 240,000 members.[65] With these numbers, the critical point is that male teachers have greater access to large numbers of teenage girls than the average man. It only takes one HIV-positive, deviant male teacher in a school that has several diligent and great male teachers to make an impact on schoolgirls' HIV rates.

In the district education offices I visited prior to school interviews, the major concern was the number of teachers dying of HIV/AIDS. The government had stopped hiring new teachers because of a strained budget and a structural-adjustment freeze in increasing the size of the public sector, and this meant that a teacher's death could have a devastating effect on a school. These challenges were reflected in the schools I visited. For example, in discussing general issues in the province at the beginning of one interview, Jerry, a boy in high school, explained:

> [Why there is] declining education in Nyanza is that you find in many schools there are not enough teachers. For example, this school, they are around only eight teachers. And these teachers, you find that one teacher can teach from Form 1 to Form 4 one subject. So it's very difficult for that teacher. They have a very big burden to do this. For example, if the teacher gets sick, who will teach that subject in school? If the teacher fell sick and they are the only teacher teaching that subject in the whole school, it is very difficult for that subject to go on. So the education will still decline. HIV/ AIDS has affected most of the teachers.

Connecting high AIDS-related mortality among teachers with schoolgirl reports of teacher-student relationships highlighted the fact that HIV was detrimental not only to youth education, but also to HIV risk among young women pursuing education.

## TWO COMPETING NORMATIVE SYSTEMS FOR GIRLS

As I have discussed thus far, transactional sex relationships were a viable and normalized option for girls in school to pursue in order to meet their needs. However, as Richard Jessor notes, "many adolescents who seem to be at high risk nevertheless do not succumb to high risk behavior, or are less involved in it than their peers, or if involved, seem to abandon it more rapidly than others."[66] Indeed, in this setting, there were many girls who did not engage in transactional relationships, and it is important to understand why, despite prevailing norms around these relationships, some girls did not succumb. Thus, even while there are several *risk* factors facilitating young women's engagement in these relationships, it is also important to account for *protective* factors, those that "moderate, buffer, insulate against, and thereby mitigate the impact of risk on adolescent behavior and development."[67]

When I examined young women's strategies for navigating through school, it became clear that their choices were a result of their grappling with two competing normative systems circulating in their school environments: a sequential model and a combination model.

The *sequential model* of proceeding through high school was the traditional model; in this model, young women were expected to sequence their expectations, consumption desires, and longings. They were to discipline them while in school and wait, privileging a focus on school and succeeding well, and putting off relationships and consumption for later.[68] The historical antecedent for this model was the increasing value placed on education, especially as a means to getting jobs that would provide income to live the good life, or *raha* (as discussed in chapter 3), which for young women meant being able to eventually participate in the kinds of consumption that met new cultural standards of beauty (chapter 4). This model was what many girls grew up hearing about at home from parents and grandparents whose own experiences growing up concretely reflected this reality and fueled their hope for and significant investment in their children and grandchildren. As detailed in chapter 3, they had seen clearly that those who went to school in the colonial and early postcolonial era were the ones who prospered, got salaried jobs, and did well. Further, this model was embodied and regularly preached by the female teachers and principals who taught them. Indeed, perhaps part of the willingness of the faculty at the schools I visited to allow me to interview their students was due to the fact that I presented a fresh example of the success of this model.[69] For them, focusing on school, going on to tertiary education (all secondary school teachers had a university degree), and then getting married and having children had placed them in exactly the position they were hoping and encouraging their female students to achieve.

By contrast, the *combination model* of proceeding through high school pushed girls to simultaneously combine relationships, school, and consumption.[70] It was the result of a profound skepticism about the sequential model. As noted earlier in this chapter, while participation in the educational system was now universal among Luo-Nyanza youth, there was increasing disillusionment about the material returns of education. Increasing numbers of youth educated through high school were at home with no jobs. In this situation, it was no longer clear whether going to school would lead to an affluent lifestyle. In this more recent model, education continued to be valuable; however, relationships with providing men were seen as an important means to both completing education and pursuing consumption. Indeed, these relationships enabled them to become—and enjoy being—the modern women that school was attempting to transform them into, school that some could not afford without providing men. The stance of parents and grandparents was ambivalence about both education and its returns. They openly and regularly discussed it as they complained about the rising costs of sending their children to school in everyday conversations with peers, which their children overheard, even as they discussed (as noted in chapter 4) their ambivalence about transactional relationships.

Both systems entailed a gamble for young women. The first model required girls to gamble that their waiting would pay off, that rejecting men for now and focusing on school would be worth it in the end. However, as I discuss in the next chapter, for many this was not the case, since the end of school resulted in a loss of family support in terms of pocket money, combined with a lack of employment or low-paying employment that severely limited their ability to accomplish their desired consumption. The second model, as illustrated in the example of Rachel, the orphan girl who was abandoned by her providing boyfriend when she got pregnant, was also a gamble. It required girls to gamble on not getting pregnant and thus on not losing both their man and their chance to complete their education. Additionally, they were also inadvertently gambling on not acquiring HIV in their pursuit of education and consumption.

Most of the chapter so far has described stories of girls who followed the combination model. In the following two case studies, I briefly describe the life stories of two girls who followed the sequential model, as they reflect on how they were able to complete their high school education amid widespread attrition among their fellow classmates, and on what they perceived as a normative environment in which the combination model supporting consumption and relationships with teachers reigned.

### Sarah: "You Don't Seem to Be Like a Girl"

Sarah was a young woman I met who was working as a librarian while waiting on the results of her final high school exams, which would determine whether she would go on to university.[71] She was the first of three girls, and clearly felt the responsibility to set a positive example for her younger siblings, one of whom was still in secondary school and the other of whom was finishing up elementary school. She came from a relatively poor family, with her mother engaged in business, while her father did seasonal work as a mechanic. She had managed to get this far in her education through a combination of merit-based scholarships and bursaries supporting her through school. The process of applying for these scholarships was stressful, as she had to apply every term—in a school system with three terms a year—and would receive about Kshs 3000 ($40) to help her through school. While most bursaries in her school were given to orphans—she estimated that about half the students in her school were single or double orphans—she was able to get them based on merit. Her hope was to do well enough to get into medical school, a bachelor's degree in Kenya, and become a doctor. In describing her story of getting this far in her education, she characterized her choices as very different from many of her fellow female students. In contrast to city-based friends who would "roam around town . . . cheat on parents, don't go to school," and who engaged themselves in "raha" and told her how "you don't know life," she deliberately chose to go to a rural school so that she would not be similarly "influenced." However, on arriving in high school, she found similar issues among her fellow female students. Indeed, at the school where she landed, they used to bring a nurse in annually to test girls for pregnancy. Girls who were found to be pregnant were "chased away from school," (though the boys who made the girls pregnant were not). The attrition due to pregnancy, a lack of school fees, and low morale because of the toughness of school among girls was high. She was one of eight girls left by her final year of high school. By all accounts, Sarah was at the top of her class, competing and keeping up with the boys, especially in science and mathematics. She used to tell her fellow female classmates to "leave makeup, hair aside and concentrate." Encouraged by the principal and teachers, she felt that one "must sacrifice yourself" in order to succeed in school. She felt that boys would often be "cheating on girls" and wasting their time, which was detrimental to their studies. She was sure to clearly define her relationship with the boys by telling them that "mine will be concerning education" and nothing else. So they would "discuss Maths, personal discussion, solve problems on the board" and engage in other such educational activities. Indeed, so focused was she on excelling in her science education that some boys would remark to her that "you don't seem to be like a girl." Sarah lived with her grandmother while going to her day school. Many teachers were concerned that she would not complete school, because grandmothers were traditionally thought to be less disciplinarian than parents since "grandmother won't follow you" and ask "where are you going?" As a result, many grandchildren, who in this setting were often orphans, would get "curious" and engage in relationships with men. The fear of students left to their own devices was particularly acute in a day school where students entered at 7:15 A.M. and left at 5 P.M., after which "the teacher doesn't follow after you; when you make a mistake, there is nowhere you can run to," especially if you lived with a grandparent. Success in school would, to a greater extent, depend on self-motivation. She credited her focus in school to her parents who had "made me be patient with myself" and told her "don't mess so that followers can do well also." Sarah was approached by a teacher for an affair in the course of high school. He asked to see her and told her to have a seat. When she asked him what was wrong, he told her that since he came to that school, he had been looking at her. He asked if he could have a friendship with her, and she said no, and told the deputy principal. Meanwhile, she described other girls as telling her, "with me, I could just allow him, to get the money." Similarly to Lizzy, other students did not understand her refusal to have a relationship with a teacher. In her case, her reporting of the teacher resulted in his being fired, and she noted, "that sir is not in school." This was the only case I heard with this outcome.

Sarah was clearly an anomaly. She was one of the rare few 8% of girls in Luo-Nyanza who had managed to complete their high school education without dropping out because of school fees, despite coming from a relatively poor family. She had also done so without getting pregnant. She was able to achieve this while living in a vulnerable position in the eyes of teachers—staying with a grandmother who would be less of a disciplinarian than parents. This achievement was not an accident. In addition to the individual ambition and will of Sarah, it is clear that several structural protective factors were at work that made her story possible. Sarah's family provided strong support both in positioning her as a role model for her sisters, and in supporting her decision to go to a rural school to pursue her education. Boys challenging her femininity reflected their dominant normative expectation that girls would follow the combination model, pursuing consumption and relationships for sex while going to school. However, Sarah was able to legitimately follow the sequential model preached by teachers. She chose to only have relationships for education, eschewing sex, the distractions of such relationships, and thus the annual risk and fear of being kicked out of school for pregnancy. And she also chose not to be a *consuming woman*, leaving aside hair and makeup in order to "concentrate" while in school. Ironically, the boys' resistance to her sequential model was probably because it was similar to the masculinity of restraint boys were constructing, as noted earlier. When girls similarly "sacrificed" and engaged in disciplined waiting, the gendered contrast and their constructed superiority were lost. This, after all, was young men's sole strategy if they stayed in school. Exposed to the same consumptive environment, and in the absence of normative transactional relationships in which they may acquire money and resources,[72] young men had the option of either dropping out of school altogether in order to pursue work, or exercising restraint and waiting.

## Ann: "Be Satisfied"

Ann, a 19-year-old, was an orphan working in a temporary job as she waited for the results of her high school exams. She was currently staying with her grandmother, who was around 80 years old. She had experienced a lot of loss in her young life, first with both of her parents dying when she was seven, and then with her first-born brother dying when she was 16. She had four living siblings left—two older and two younger. She credited her two older brothers with pushing her to finish high school, and she was hoping to follow in their footsteps and go on to university. She wanted to study journalism. Girls, she thought, did well academically "when being followed" because girls were "more distracted in school." She felt that part of this was because boys were valued more than girls. In her words, "people say that boys should be valued more; they feel that girls can get married at any time and bring them the [bride] wealth." She estimated that only one-sixth of the girls she graduated elementary school with finished high school. She felt that when their families could not pay school fees, girls were sent home, and during the time they were at home, they could "mess up." Many of her schoolmates in elementary school dropped out because of pregnancy and a lack of school fees. She herself had been able to finish, but still had a big balance of fees to pay off at her high school. Many former classmates were at home, had gotten married, or had children—situations that, especially in the last two cases, meant the end of education. In her case, part of what was underlying her getting as far as she did in education despite similar school-fee challenges was the things she said to herself to stay disciplined. She would tell herself to be content and "don't look around at others," "plan with the little you have," "know to carry yourself around," "be satisfied," and there is a "time for everything."

Ann had had a particularly difficult journey in her young life. A double orphan living with her grandmother, she represented an even rarer example of a female high school graduate. Orphan girls were particularly vulnerable to dropping out of school.[73] Ann, despite the high dropout rate of her classmates, had been able to stay focused on school despite these challenges. In a way similar to Sarah's story, a key structural protective factor was the strong family support from her brothers, both as role models and in pushing her to stay in school and to finish. In addition, her final statements are striking in describing explicit mantras in line with the sequential normative model and what many female teachers preached to their students: to avoid becoming a consuming woman until she could afford it. Thus, delayed gratification, avoiding peer comparisons, and being content and satisfied with what she had were strategies she pursued in order to manage her relative poverty and the prevailing normative environment urging consumption.

The cases of Sarah and Ann illustrate the challenges of remaining in school for young women in this setting. In addition to high individual motivation and willpower, their avoiding consumption was enabled by parental and family support—both financial and emotional[74]—and depended on a school-sanctioned sequential model urging them to wait and focus on school first. For Sarah, it was staying away from makeup and being content with simple hair, and for Ann, it was being content and satisfied with what she had and delaying gratification until later. For both, the hope was that education might one day yield the things they wanted. Indeed, when I met Sarah, for example, she had a perm in her hair and was fashionably dressed. Clearly, after graduation, and with a temporary job, she was now able to spend some money on "being a girl" in a manner intelligible not just to Luo-Nyanzans, but to girls everywhere: that is, being a consuming woman who did her hair and wore makeup. They both also saw boys and relationships as distractions from the task of school. Involvement with boys would mess up their professional hopes. The evidence for this was all around them, with dramatic attrition rates for their female schoolmates, which served as a cautionary tale. This was also part of the sequential model, preached by many adults, as illustrated in the epigraph opening this chapter. The idea that "boys will destroy your life" was a widespread part of the messages to school-going girls. The sequential model, as briefly noted earlier, also follows a striking parallel to the model implicitly followed by young men to avoid HIV, discussed in chapter 4. For them, avoiding expensive women inadvertently meant avoiding HIV. For young women here, staying away from boys and men and postponing consumption and modernity also meant staying away from HIV.

## CONCLUSION

Despite the high HIV-prevalence rates in this setting, most young women are not HIV positive. However, this chapter illustrates the difficulty and challenges that girls face when navigating through school without "messing up" by getting "a child or a disease." For the unfortunate proportion who got HIV, social structure and individual agency came together to create a fatal situation. At the individual level, schoolgirls were moved to search for money in ways that increased their HIV risk, moved by perceived gendered necessities presented during the course of pursuing their education—necessities that were beyond the means of their parents or guardians. A boyfriend with money was a more likely source of income than poor parents who did not see the things they wanted as "needs." A number of structural factors also facilitated young women's risk. While school would appear to be precisely the context in which HIV risk is mitigated, there were a number of ways in which the opposite was true. The social structure of school reinforced norms about the things that were considered needs that required consumption, and norms of engaging in transactional relationships with working-class men to get money to pay for those needs. (Ironically, these relationships sometimes also resulted in the end of school if girls became pregnant.) It did this through structuring the setting in which large groups of young women met, and through shaping the dynamics occurring within those groups. The structure of the school calendar played a role in releasing girls from school on a timetable that coincided with the increased availability of men with money in their hometowns. Finally, the risk was not just outside of the school context, but also within. The potentially widespread nature of relationships with teachers meant that school was not always a safe place for young women, but was in fact precisely the place in which HIV could be acquired.

Two key facts suggest that this experience was not unique to the Luo of Nyanza. First, the increasing feminization of HIV rates in sub-Saharan Africa suggests a model of smaller pools of men infecting large numbers of women, and further suggests the role of generation and gender in increasing risk for young women throughout Africa. Schools structurally create small but dense sexual networks in which one new infection can spark a miniepidemic with great speed.[75] Secondly, the widespread nature of transactional relationships and their being described as occurring in school settings in particular in several accounts from across the continent also suggest that this is significant not just for young Luo women, but also for young women in other parts of sub-Saharan Africa. A key social structure that brings increasing numbers of young women into contact with older men with access to money and resources is school. The embedded nature of school in many local communities across the continent—not just as a source of education and knowledge, but also as a source of income and business—means that relationships between teachers and students provide an entanglement that makes sanctions difficult. Thus, it is likely that the school structure and its links to the production of gendered disparities in HIV rates among youth in Luo-Nyanza are being replicated in other settings in sub-Saharan Africa.

In the next chapter, I consider what happened when consuming young women produced in school transitioned into the workforce. In particular, I examine the challenges many faced in getting access to their own income to meet their needs as they encountered and navigated a third social structure—gendered labor markets. The chapter illustrates how, in similar ways to school, the pursuit of employment complicated young women's attempts to stay HIV free.

# 6 Gendered Economies and the Role of Ecology in HIV Risk

> According to me, for us as women . . . the main problem is income for us to do anything. There is lack of income.
>
> Jane, young out-of-school woman

> They are jobless. Ladies are jobless.
>
> Henry, young out-of-school man

The obvious solution to consuming women's challenge of meeting continual needs requiring consumption of modern goods seems to be for them to find or create jobs to earn their own money. However, in this chapter, I unpack a final startling paradox and examine why women who work have higher rates of HIV. The chapter begins with a discussion of how young women transitioning out of school and into the labor force confronted a gendered economic structure—gendered in access to jobs and, as a result, gendered in access to income. Economies are gendered when they structure occupations in gendered ways. That is, factors such as access to work (who can work and where), the division of labor within work (occupational sex segregation), and compensation (pay) for particular kinds of work often differ by gender and often do so in ways that disadvantage women.[1] In the case of compensation, for example, as noted in chapter 2, women are paid less than men, even in the most advanced global economies and despite antidiscrimination legislation. The gendered nature of economies and, in particular, the imbalance in women's access to the fruits of their labor are important in this case because economic realities structure intimate relationships and sexual economies.[2] In particular, the predominantly one-way transfer of money and gifts—from men to women—in transactional relationships reflects the fact that in most settings, men have relatively greater access to money and resources due to the gendered structure of local economies.[3] This economic reality, as I will show, had particular implications for young women in and out of school in Nyanza province, who are produced as consuming women and are trying to find money to pay for needs that require continual replenishment. I illustrate how this was consequential for young women by showing the gap between income and needs, as well as why young women's access to the labor market, in some ways *exacerbated* their HIV risk. In the final section of the chapter, I use the specific example of fishing, a major industry in Nyanza province, to show how its gendered economy and the ecological changes in and around Lake Victoria, the largest freshwater lake in Africa, combined to exacerbate young women's HIV risk.

## THE SCHOOL-TO-WORK TRANSITION

For many African youth, the transition from school to work is gradual, often beginning with part-time, unpaid work when they are children going to school, followed by a gradual shift to paid work as they grow older. Some of this income goes toward funding their education. The transition out of full-time education is also sometimes gradual, with full-time work during the day and part-time vocational courses in the evenings and on weekends.[4] For young Luo women, the transition out of school and into work was elongated and characterized by ambivalence and uncertainty, and this made it a difficult period for many. The exit from school often came after several months or years of an interrupted education. One term in school was followed by a term at home while waiting for fees to be collected from family and relatives to pay for another school term or year. Eventually the will to keep searching for money, the piling up of unpaid school debt, or simply the end of school fees' availability led to a dropout or termination of education at the end of high school, with no money to pay for higher education. Because of this situation, many young women left school involuntarily and continued long afterward to yearn to return, if given an opportunity. For example, Akinyi, who participated in a youth group, shared her story:

AKINYI:  I finished Form 4 but conceived in the process so I went for my [final high school] exams when I was already having a baby. The main problem that brings this is lack of school fees, maybe your parent is unable, and maybe you can't afford school fees when you are sent home, and so you turn back to men. So that is why I didn't do well in school and that is why I can't get a better job.

SANYU:  So were you sent home for fees a lot during school?

AKINYI:  Yes. Even up to now I am still having a huge balance. I sat for my exams in 2000 [six years ago]. I am still having interest in school. The only thing is school fees. Even up to now I can still go back, I am still young.

Akinyi's story captures not only the barrier of school fees for poor families, but also how many young women's journeys through school became entangled with relationships with "working-class" men who promised help with school fees. In her case, despite the pregnancy, she was able to be among the rare few to graduate high school, but she was not able to do as well as she otherwise would have and was unable to carry on with her education.

As noted in the previous chapter, despite the government relief of school fees, while over 93% of Kenyans and all Luo-Nyanzans begin primary school, over 80% and 90%, respectively, do not complete high school. In the 1980s, responding to large-scale attrition at the time, the Kenyan government revamped the primary school (grades 1 through 8) syllabus to include the provision of prevocational education. This shift placed increased emphasis on agriculture and craft skills such as carpentry and tailoring, as well as on business studies that would enable students to set up their own businesses once they left school. However, by the time youth reached secondary school, their parents' and their own aspirations had stretched to the expectation of white-collar jobs. As Eisemon and Schwille noted: "Parents do not send their children to school to become better farmers or to learn vernacular languages and practical skills that will suit them for rural life. They want an education for their children that affords them an opportunity for a much better life off the farm."[5] The point of school was to become educated, to become modern.[6] Youth themselves felt that "an educated person cannot work in the *shamba* [farm]."[7] Going as far as secondary school and then ending up in the field doing agricultural work seemed like a negation of the past several years of struggle, hard work, and identity transformation.

In every high school I visited, I asked students what their job aspirations were. Typical answers were to become a doctor, a lawyer, a journalist,
or a teacher—all occupations that required postsecondary education, as
opposed to starting their own business, for example, which did not.
Implied in these aspirations were the status and the affluent lifestyle that
these professional occupations would afford, with stable income, a nice
house, the ability to decorate it nicely, and perhaps a car. For young women
in particular, a professional job would lend itself to financial independence from their parents and husbands. Conversations about the ideal age
of marriage were often coupled with the need to be financially independent before they got married, "so that you don't depend on the man so
much." They feared that dependence might make them vulnerable to
domestic violence. "Some may even start beating you. If you don't even
have a job, where you will go to?" The problem with these aspirations was
that the path for many of them to achieve their goals was very constrained,
and they would likely be unable to achieve them, as the youth out of school
just ahead of them were slowly realizing. This was true even in merit-
based schools that only admitted the smartest students in Nyanza province. In one such school I visited, for example, only three students out of a
graduating class of 150 received high enough grades to qualify for a government-sponsored university place. Everyone else would have to pay out
of pocket to attend one of the many burgeoning private educational estab-
lishments. Despite these sorts of results being replicated year after year in
schools across the province, the dream of university or continuing on with
education continued to dominate the plans of youth in secondary school
for the future. Margaret Frye has argued that in the case of school girls in
Malawi, the continued disjuncture between aspirations to professional
careers and the reality that very few in fact achieved them suggests less an
irrational imagined future and more an assertion of a particular kind of
moral identity, marking those girls who held these aspirations as superior
to girls who had dropped out of school, and setting them apart as perse-
vering, determined young women able to resist boys and focus on their
education.[8] In this setting, while this seemed part of the story, the shock,
disillusionment, and disappointment of the job market when they
attempted to enter it suggested that there was also an ignorance of the
reality: that is, either they lacked an awareness of the structural reality of

the job market, or they had a sense that this structural reality would not apply to them.

In looking at the survey data, the jobs youth wanted did not match the jobs they ended up doing. The Kenya Demographic and Health Survey (KDHS) from 2010 shows that the most common types of jobs among Kenyan women under 30 who reported that they were currently working were being an employee or self-employed in agricultural work (17%) and professional/technical or management work (12%). Young women also did sales (4.6%), skilled manual labor (4.2%), and household/domestic work (3.7%). These trends were similar among Luo-Nyanza women, with the most common occupations being agriculture (18%), professional/ technical or management work (14%), sales (6%), skilled manual labor (5%), and household/domestic work (3.5%). Similarly, among men under 30, the most common types of jobs among those reporting that they were currently working were being an employee or self-employed in agricultural work (34.4%) and professional/technical or management work (12.1%). Young men also did unskilled manual labor (10.8%) and sales (6.3%). Among Luo-Nyanza men, the most common occupations were agriculture (30.4%), unskilled manual labor (18.8%), skilled manual labor (8.5%), and professional/technical or management work (7.5%). Given that 36% and 42% of young Kenyan women and men (30% and 38% for Luo-Nyanza women and men) had at least some high school education, these statistics suggest that few were able to secure the kinds of professional jobs to which they aspired. However, the problem for young women who had transitioned out of school was much more basic than a mismatch between job aspirations set in school and economic realities once they left. Getting a job—any job—was a challenge compared to young men.

## A GENDERED ECONOMY

From the perspective of young people, access to jobs was clearly gendered. Young men and women were in general agreement that while girls had almost no options for work while going to school, boys had plenty. Perceived gendered disparity in needs, illustrated in the previous chapter, was exacerbated by a perceived gendered disparity in access to jobs to meet those needs. In several focus group discussions, I asked girls whether there were ways for them to earn money, and they said that their parents and extended family were the only source, and that they could not work for money and go to school at the same time. Initially unconvinced, I pursued this further after girls noted that there were few or no options for girls. The following excerpt is from one such interview in a focus group among schoolgirls. I first asked them if there were ways boys could earn money. After listing them, they proceeded to explain why each of these jobs was not appropriate or accepted for women to do:

SANYU: If there are no other ways for girls to earn money other than what their parents give, then what about boys, do they have a chance to earn money?

GRACE: Yes.

SANYU: Even in school, like what things can they do?

GRACE: Boys can make even charcoal.

MARY: They can go to the lake to fish.

HARRIET: They can do the job of *boda boda* [bicycle taxi] on Sundays to get money.

AMOSI: During weekends, we have our weekends on Sundays, so you know some boys will have some jobs in the farm, you know people are planting, so go there and they have some jobs and when they are finishing the job, they get money.

SANYU: And girls can't do those things? *[Silent negating gestures.]*

SANYU: No? You've never seen a girl, like, make charcoal?

GRACE: It's hard work for a girl to cut a tree and make into smaller pieces for charcoal. That one is a very difficult job for a girl. *[Laughter.]*

SANYU: And girls don't fish?

AMOSI: Ah, we don't go out with that job.

SANYU: And girls don't do *boda boda?*

AMOSI: Yes.

SANYU: And they don't work on farms?

RACHEL: They work, like planting. They can go and plant, it's when they are being paid.

SANYU: How much would you be paid after a day?

RACHEL: 50 shillings [less than $1].

SANYU:  50 shillings?

RACHEL:  And it is a very big portion. *[Laughter.]*

These views were corroborated by the schoolboys I interviewed. In a typical remark, George noted, "So on that issue of the kind of jobs that they can do, here we don't have jobs that girls can do. Let's say like breaking concrete, you see, breaking concrete you cannot find a lady or a girl sitting on a concrete, splitting concrete. Things like maybe going to dig someone's garden, it's very rare for ladies to go there, and bicycle taxi, it's very rare to see a lady riding a bicycle." The suggestion of women riding the *boda boda* (bicycle taxi) or making charcoal generated a lot of laughter in my interviews with young men. Overall, it became clear in interviews that both young men and young women felt that girls would have to cross gender lines and face mockery if they were seen doing these jobs. Sheer desperation, it seems, would characterize this subversion. In the case of agricultural work, it seemed that it was less about the physical capability of women and more about the fact that young women did not want to do such jobs because they were seen as incompatible with their status as educated women.

In examining the KDHS 2010 data on age-specific rates of Kenyan and Luo-Nyanza youth currently working, it appears that the gendered labor market young people perceived was reflected in the statistics. Figure 12 suggests stark gender differences in who reported currently working (the survey specifically excluded their own residential domestic housework).[9] Overall, fewer Kenyan women (43%) under age 30 reported currently working, compared to same-aged young men (78%). Strikingly, among teenagers, three times as many young men (60%) were working compared to same-aged young women (19%). This is even though school attrition was greater for women than it was for men (see chapter 5). Women's working rates at age 25–29 were equivalent to men's working rates at age 15–19. This likely meant that, among youth who had dropped out of school, more girls were out of the formal labor force than boys. We see similar trends when we focus on Luo-Nyanza youth, though the gender differences are less stark: 29% of teenage women were currently working, compared to 46% of same-aged men. Overall, about half of young Kenyan women (43%) and Luo-Nyanza women (47%) were working, while about two-thirds of similar young men reported that they were currently working. In

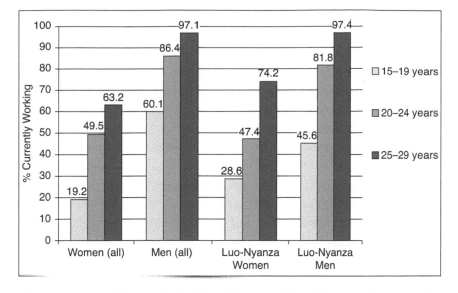

*Figure 12.* Age-specific rates (%) of those Kenyan and Luo-Nyanza youth, 15–29, who are currently working. Source: KDHS 2010.

sum, fewer young women were working than same-aged young men, even though their perceived and continual needs and expenses were greater.[10]

Educational attainment was clearly linked to current working status. Overall, women with no education reported the lowest rates of current work, compared to same-aged women at different educational levels. Women at higher levels of education, especially by age 25–29, when most were likely to have completed school, reported higher levels of current work. Overall, there seemed to be a workplace penalty for no education, and a positive premium for higher postsecondary education, with little variation among young women in the middle. Going to university or other kinds of postsecondary educational institutions provided a critical advantage in the labor market.[11] However, very few (6.9% and 2.7% among Kenyan and Luo-Nyanza women, respectively) attained higher education by age 29.[12] These few were among either the very smart who were able to secure one of the few merit-based government-sponsored university places, or the wealthy and well-connected who were able to afford self-sponsored university or vocational college places. Vocational colleges included full-time polytechnics and teacher-training colleges for those who missed university but got high enough grades to meet college standards and had family, providing men, or other sponsors who could pay for them to go. The reality for the remaining 90% of young women was that they had lower employment and thus earning rates than Kenyan men. Among 25–29-year-old Kenyan men, rates of current work varied little by educational attainment. Virtually all worked (97%). Education mattered more for the type of work they did, with less-educated men engaged more in agriculture and unskilled and skilled manual labor, while those with higher levels of education were involved in professional/technical and management work. These trends were similar among Luo-Nyanza men. These data begin to paint a picture of the gendered job market girls emerging from high school were confronting, and the potential implications for their ability to provide for themselves, given their disproportionate needs compared to men. Indeed, this implicitly set them up to be dependent on providing men in intimate relationships or in their family to an even greater extent than boys, who had fewer needs and more financial means.

## THE STRUGGLE OF THE TRANSITION

For both young men and young women, the period after exiting school was characterized by disillusionment as well as a reassessment and a recalibration of expectations as they came to terms with the fact that they were likely not going to be able to achieve their dream of going on with their education, at least in the near term. They had to adjust to a more practical orientation to working life after high school, which was often difficult.[13] However, while, as I show, the struggles were *discursively* similar, as the data illustrate, men's transition into work outside the home was ultimately more successful in terms of finding a job than that of young women.

### Young Men

Young men's concerns were less about *no work* and more about the *kind* of work they were doing, regardless of the amount of education they had received. Several young men, for example, talked about the challenge of certification. Certification, which reflects completion of particular educational goals, was especially important in trying to find a job, since it was used by employers as a way of deciding among many applicants. Certificates from school reflect national examination grades as opposed to the number of years of school. As a result, certificates are only given after passing the elementary school exam (Kenya Certificate of Primary Education [Grade 8]) or after passing the high school exam (Kenya Certificate of Secondary Education [Form 4]). Youth who dropped out before completing elementary school or high school were thus at a particular disadvantage.[14] Thus, while daily wage jobs such as slashing grass or doing agricultural work in someone's garden were possible to get, more permanent, salaried jobs needed a high school diploma. In a typical description of this struggle, Jacob, a young man, said, "Right now I have tried looking for jobs even though I am not through with my course. They want two certificates: a Form Four certificate and then one for my course. So I find it very difficult because I only have a Class Eight certificate."

As a result, his vocational school course without the high school certificate resulted in a struggle on the job market. Much of what made this a lengthy process was the fact that many youth faced a no-win situation of needing experience in order to get a job but not having people willing to give them paid work experience in order to qualify. Another young man, Ezekiel, described his struggle to get a job as a driver: "I have a driving license [and] have tried looking for jobs in different companies. You are told to produce a Form Four certificate, and that you need to have five years of experience, but I only have three years of experience, so I can't get a job." As a result, he was having to do other jobs, including shaving hair, to make a living while he waited out the years. Because only having a single job yielded little money, many young men juggled multiple smaller jobs in order to make ends meet. In some settings, for example, young men would fish at night and do *boda boda* taxi work during the day. Engaging in "multiple livelihoods" to generate income was a way to diversify and deal with the unpredictability of the job economy.[15]

Young men engaged in many types of jobs, and I discuss some of the main ones I encountered here. Perhaps as a consequence of my fieldwork requiring me to travel long distances on a daily basis, I encountered many young men in the transportation business. For example, I often talked with a young taxi driver in his mid-20s, Zacchaeus, who had stopped school at Form 1 because he did not have money for school fees to continue further. One of his brothers had a car, so he learned to drive and eventually got a job working for a man his brother knew who owned six taxis and ran a taxi service at the airport. This is, in fact, how I met him. This was a really good job, as jobs for young men went. He had held it for three years and was earning Kshs 6,000 ($86) a month. Since rent cost him only Kshs 1,500 ($21) a month, he had a relatively large amount of disposable income compared to his peers. However, there were also a lot of demands on his income since two of his brothers and their wives had died of HIV, leaving behind ten orphans. He was now responsible for taking care of everyone and lamented to me that "there are so many needs, and everyone is asking for money." We can see here how a young man who would have done really well on his own, with his small nuclear family of a wife and a six-year-old child, had a large responsibility as a key provider to his extended family from an early stage in his life.[16] Other, less economically fortunate young men in the transportation business ran bicycle-taxi services (*boda boda* men). Their biographies were similar; they dropped out of school, often in elementary school or at the end of it, because there was no money to pay for secondary school. Demand for *boda boda* men across the province was high, since many villages and schools were off the main roads and the only access to them was by walking or bicycle taxi. There was also a business for men in transporting goods by bicycle, though this was highly taxing work for relatively little pay. (See figure 13.)

Young men who lived high up in plateau areas of the province where there were a lot of rocks were often involved in construction work, making concrete and bricks. Christopher described how work competed with education: "Another thing is in this area you find that young people are making concrete ... if someone drop[s] out of school, and he marries when still young, he makes concrete at least to boost his life or the family. So it's very difficult and uphill on the plateau. They [also] have brick making. So you find that many young people are dropping out of school to go and make bricks."

Some young men who lived near the lake engaged in agriculture, farming small gardens by the lake and selling the produce in the local markets, or fishing. One young man's career trajectory, however, led him back to school at a teacher's training college. Crispin completed his high school

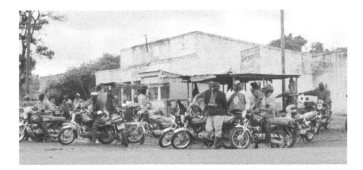

*Figure 13. Boda boda* men. Photograph by Jackson Wanga.

with the encouragement of his older brother, who was the only permanently employed person in his village. He did fairly well in his high school exams, but did not pursue university; he instead went to the city to do contract work for a year, but was soon frustrated by this. He then returned to the village and began small jobs such as burning charcoal and collecting sand (for construction). When he had saved Kshs 1000, he used this as capital to start a shopkeeping business. His high school certification allowed him to do freelance work in data collection with the national census bureau, as well as with the electoral commission, which gave him additional capital to aid his business. He started selling slippers and branched into ladies footwear, which was in high demand. He then got married, and, at the time of the interview, had two children. He said he returned to school at the age of 30 to become a teacher because his friends had said that, while anyone could do business, not everyone had the opportunity to return to school and become a professional. The status of having a profession, aspired to by so many during high school, outweighed the greater amount of money he might make running his business. In sum, for most young men, finding a job was not perceived as a problem if they were willing to take on any job, even if it was not commensurate with their education.

*Young Women*

For young women, the challenge was not just the often fruitless and frustrating search for work, but also a concomitant dramatic decline in access to resources to meet their needs after school was over. Jane described her experience of postsecondary disillusionment:

> Me, I finished school in 2004 and till now I am just surviving as far as prob-
> lem is concerned. When I was in school, I could have some pocket money
> when I come back, buying my clothes, but nowadays it is upon you to strug-
> gle and get them. And you know that when we are still in school, then they
> do give us some promises, that "when you finish then I will do you this and
> this" but when you are out, the promises are there but they are nowhere to
> be seen. And then it is upon you to keep on asking, "Daddy, you said you will
> do this and that." So you will keep on reminding him and he will tell you he
> will do [it]. It is upon you to give up. So the parents, they do give us prom-
> ises but they don't fulfill them.

It is worth reiterating that the "just surviving" she discussed in the two years since she left school was not for basic needs such as food and shelter, but for pocket money and new or secondhand clothing, as highlighted in chapter 4 and 5. Support from parents and relatives while going to school— with money for school fees, a school uniform, textbooks, and pocket money (which some schools mandated)—ended once school was done. Relatives who might feel obligated to support a brother's son or a cousin's daughter through school would feel their duty was fulfilled once that child left school. For young women, as a result, the disparities between perceived needs and access to income from parents and relatives to meet those needs grew ever wider once they left school. The option for most girls was to try to find jobs, even if low paying, to address at least some of their needs, or to recalibrate their needs and be content with the little they had.

About half (47%) of the young Luo-Nyanza women surveyed reported working outside the home. This statistical reality was reflected in my field-work, where I found an even mix of young women with no paid employ-ment and young women working in a variety of low-income and itinerant jobs. These jobs included being house helpers, bar girls, and food kiosk ladies; fetching firewood and selling it; hairdressing; and selling second-hand clothes. If they were in an urban area, some were also assistants at photocopying stalls, or they ran stalls selling pay-as-you go scratch cards for mobile phones. (See figure 14, figure 15, and figure 16.)

These were "small small jobs," to use their term; rarely were they the jobs they had aspired to do. Further, even these could be hard to find or

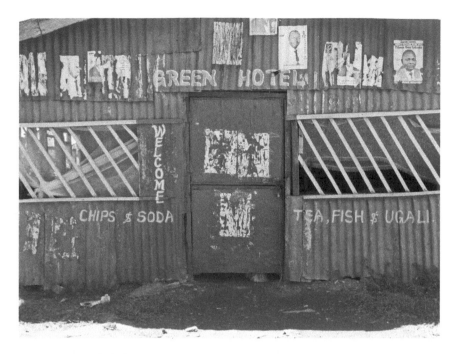

*Figure 14.* Roadside hotel. Photograph by Jackson Wanga.

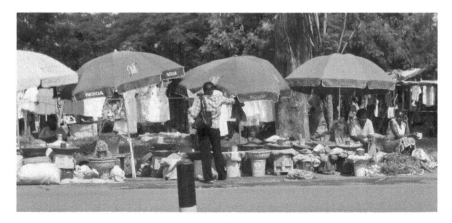

*Figure 15.* Roadside selling. Photograph by Jackson Wanga.

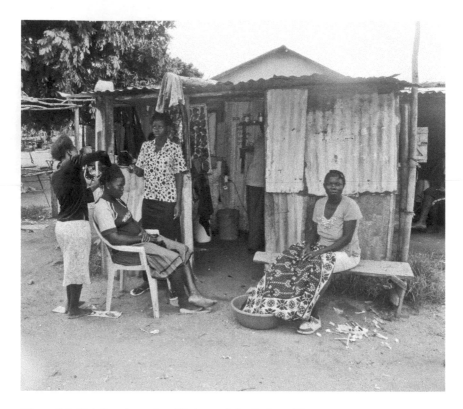

*Figure 16.* Hairdressing salon. Photograph by Jackson Wanga.

start up and paid very little money, especially relative to the needs of the young women. It was hard for many to stretch what they earned to meet and sustain the ideal life of a consuming woman with continual consumption needs. Something had to give: their perception of what counted as needs or their means of getting money.

Amanda, who was 21 years old, was an orphan taken in by a kind aunt. She graduated high school and was able to enroll in secretarial college. However, the money for fees ran out, and she had to drop out. Eventually, funding became available and she was able to join a commercial college and complete her training. However, a year after completing postsecondary education, she was still unable to find a white-collar job. She was now planting vegetables by the riverbank, which she then sold at one of the local markets. She was selling her produce for Kshs 5 or 10 shillings each, and on a good day could make as much as 200 shillings ($2.86). Her story shows that, even though she was able to gain postsecondary vocational training, she was unable to find a white-collar job, and in the end was doing a job she could have done if she had never gone to school. However, this to her was a better alternative than being unemployed or continuing a fruitless search for a professional job as a secretary.

A group of four resourceful girls also decided to strike out on their own and start a small roadside shack hotel, a small structure made of corrugated iron where customers could go in, order food, and sit at wooden tables and on plastic chairs or wooden benches. Each girl contributed Kshs 75 ($1) each, and they collectively borrowed the remaining capital they needed to buy cooking utensils and food to get started. At the time of my interview with two of the girls, the business had been running for four months with just the two of them still involved. However, even with this resourcefulness, there remained challenges:

SANYU:   So the money you get from work when you are working, or the one you get from your family, is it enough to buy like food and rent where you are staying?

RASPA:   Not enough.

SANYU:   So how do you make sure that, how do you, like, find the rest of the money?

LESI:   The first thing is that we are still staying with our parents and so we don't pay rent, and food we don't provide. But we can just give something if we feel like giving but it is not a must. So we just have to find money for personal maintenance.

For these 21-year-old young women, while they had basic provisions of food and shelter from their parents, the little money they were making had to cover all their "personal maintenance." This phrase would cover things like toiletries such as soap, deodorant, and sanitary pads.

Many other young women, however, were unemployed after a frustrating attempt to move forward with their education. The following are a few excerpts from three different young women who were living at home:

BELINDA:   Well I did my Form 4 in the year 2004 . . . and my dad told me that he will take me to any course that I chose and I told him . . . I just wanted to do these medical courses. . . . There was a recruitment [for a job that had on-the-job training] and he told me that he didn't have the backdoor money and then I asked him, "What backdoor money do these people want?" And there was no feedback and then I just kept quiet. We are just there with him.

BETTY: I did my KCPE in 2000, then the year 2001, I went to study hairdressing in Eldoret [a town]. I finished and worked for six months. After that, I returned home and have not returned there. Now I am just at home. [With your parents?] Yes, my dad.

LISA: Me, I did my KCPE in 2000. Since then, I have just been at home with my mother. My father died.

In the first example, Belinda's father was unable to come up with the bribe (backdoor money) needed to ensure his daughter's place in the job. The need for a bribe was an indicator of how high the demand was for such positions. Since that incident, she had been at home for two years. Betty and Lisa had been unemployed and at home for most of the five years after finishing primary school (KCPE).

Girls who did not have paid work were often characterized or would characterize themselves as "at home," "just there," "idle," or "sitting at home." These devaluing phrases belied the large amount of invaluable and indispensable unpaid labor they engaged in. Indeed, the substantial amount of domestic work they did was precisely because they were now permanently home from school and had no "excuse" such as school homework or a job outside the home. This work included caring for younger siblings or their own children, cooking "from scratch" for the extended family living in the household, cleaning both in and around the house, searching for water because of the severe lack of piped water in many communities, hand-washing and ironing (with a charcoal-powered iron) laundry for multiple household members, engaging in subsistence farming, and so on. This was very exhausting work that could engage them from early morning until late evening with little free time, a point I will return to later in the chapter.

Living at home with no paid work was difficult not just physically, but also emotionally. Jeanette, who was 22 years old and lived in an informal settlement with her mother, was the sixth of seven children. While in high school, she met a man who was her sister's neighbor and worked in immigration services in a border town, and they started dating. Unfortunately, she got pregnant while in Form 3 at the age of 17 and returned home to deliver. Tragedy struck soon after when her father and one of what turned out to be twins both died around the same time. The double loss and contemplating what it would be like to leave her surviving child while she went back to school made her decide to stay at home. She did not have a job or a way of earning her own money. So she said that she was just, as she put it, "sitting idle," which she found hard. She was in many ways in limbo—she did not want to marry the father of her child because her now deceased father had not approved, she did not want to leave her child at home while she went back to school, and she did not have a job outside the home and was thus financially dependent on her mother. Since she sometimes helped out at her mother's tailoring shop, she was contemplating following in her footsteps and could see a path out of her present predicament.

## LABOR MARKET TO THE RESCUE?

At the outset, it would seem that young women who are not engaging in paid employment and thus have little or no independent money would be most at risk for relationships with older men with money and thus for acquiring HIV. However, when we examine the DHS data and look at the prevalence of HIV rates by employment status, we find the *opposite* to be true. Among Kenyan women, young women (age 15–29) who work for pay have HIV rates roughly *twice* as high (9%) as women who do not work for pay (4.1%). Similarly, among Luo-Nyanza women, paid workers have HIV rates just over twice as high (29.2%) as those who do not work for pay (13.1%). These trends are statistically significant.[17] These results are startling and counterintuitive, because if a lack of money is really at the heart of young women's HIV rates, then jobs that give them access to their own money should reduce their likelihood of engaging in relationships in which they are financially dependent.

Indeed, several intervention programs in this vein have attempted to set up small-scale programs enabling young women to earn their own money through microcredit to start small businesses.[18] Young women themselves assumed that working for pay was the answer to HIV prevention. The following is an excerpt from a focus group interview with young women in vocational school:

SANYU:   So what about women, what kind of prevention, do you think practically would work among women?

RACHEL:  Abstinence.

MARY:   If you get married to one faithful partner.

PRISCA:  And no money? *[Someone laughs.]*

RACHEL:  Now we resort to this practical work, like manual job, like if you're so poor, you go to somebody's *shamba,* at least look for a way of earning a living.

MARY:   But who will do agree to do that?

RACHEL:  You can be a house girl, start your own *jua kali* [artisanal work] things, or cooperatives at home, or merry-go-rounds.[19] Just indulge in these women affair things like meetings, you can also go and make bricks, construct, at least make something that makes you busy. You know some women, if you can at least have your daily bread, this money, you won't go embarrassing these men. You only go for these men because of lack of money.

The comments between Rachel and Mary are interesting. Rachel's suggestions were all norm-breaking: first that educated girls should go back to farm work, which Mary questions, and then that women should engage in work traditionally done by men (*jua kali,* making bricks, and construction), if things were that bad, in order to get money. The logic was clear: young women engage in these relationships because of money; so if women worked for their own money, they would not need to engage in these relationships. However, it would seem from the prevalence rates that the apparent solution to the problem of girls' needs—being able to work to earn their own money to pay for their own needs—does not necessarily bring an end to or reduce HIV risk, but might in fact exacerbate it.

What appears as a paradox, however, becomes less so when we connect it to earlier findings. As noted in chapter 2, young women under 30 living in wealthier households have higher rates of HIV. To the extent that part of this wealth is their own, the findings concerning work and HIV here are another reflection of this relationship. As the findings in this chapter so far suggest, young women who stayed home and did not earn independent income were forced to recalibrate their needs in light of limited resources and be satisfied with what their parents or husbands could provide. They were also more likely to have demanding domestic housework schedules, as well as relatively limited opportunities to meet working-class men outside their home. Thus, they were less able or indeed unable to continue being consuming women. Many simply, by and large, opted out of being a consuming woman.

Henry, a young man, expressed what very few seemed to dispute:

> And for ladies, for you to have something to do for you to earn money, at least it takes some years. Now these boys will be getting money and trying to lure them because they are jobless, ladies are jobless. Now easily most of them will be going for those men or boys who have got money. Now the majority will be running for those men who have got money. And some men also they don't have that money so they that will not be going for those ladies. Because ladies will be *always* after money. If you don't have money, no room for you. (my emphasis)

Henry noted how much harder it was for young women to find jobs and also how their lack of jobs was driving them into the arms of men with money. However, something to pay particular attention to in his statement is that "ladies will be *always* after money." Arguably, it is the *continual* nature of women's need for money that is the problem. As shown in chapter 5, in pursuing their education, young women were also being produced as modern young women, and to be modern was to engage in practices of consumption that marked their difference from traditional village girls. While the modern things boys wanted were one-time items (a bicycle or a radio cassette, for example), young women wanted things that needed continual replenishing (sanitary pads, Vaseline, makeup, and so on). They had to be continual consumers and thus continual transactors. Creating a constant need for consumption is the point of a consuming culture—to constantly cultivate in subjects desires requiring consumption that are, ideally, never satisfied, thus keeping customers coming back for more. Young women who went to work had less incentive to recalibrate their needs; they were earning an independent income. However, because of the low-income jobs they were finding, young women who did not recalibrate experienced continual frustration and struggle because the "small

small" money they earned would never be enough to keep up with their needs. The remaining option for young women in this position was to find a providing boyfriend to supplement their income and underwrite their expenses.

This project was enabled by the new structural environment that young women who worked were in and the stage of life they were in since having left school. Moving from the structure of school to the structure of work moved them outside the purview of relatives, gave them relative freedom, and presented a lot more autonomy, mobility, and opportunities to meet providing men, who were, it was hoped, also potential husbands. Being able to remain a consuming woman meant that such a young woman could continue to maintain local, modern standards of beauty and attractiveness, an especially important goal in the postschooling, husband-hunting years. Unfortunately, providing men—slightly older, wealthier men—were also more likely to have higher rates of HIV, as illustrated in chapter 4.

In the next section I turn to examining how the dynamics of a gendered economy structured HIV risk for young working women in Nyanza province by focusing on a particular industry. Specifically, I show how the gendered structure of the fishing economy, an industry that employed many young people in Nyanza, along with a changing ecological environment in and around Lake Victoria, exacerbated HIV risk for young working women.

## A GENDERED ECONOMY AND HIV RISK

### The Socioecological Setting of the Lake

The most dominant geographic feature of Nyanza province is Lake Victoria, the second largest freshwater body in the world and the source of the River Nile. Throughout my fieldwork, as I moved between districts, I discovered how much of Luoland hugs Lake Victoria, how much life was organized around the lake, and how dependent on the lake many Luo were. This discovery was emphasized by an event I encountered midway through research. One afternoon, on arrival in Homa Bay, a major lakeside town in the southern part of Nyanza province, a big convention was underway at

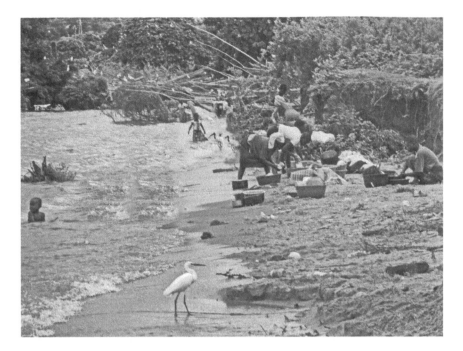

*Figure 17.* Multiple uses of the lake. Photograph by Jackson Wanga.

the hotel where I was staying. The event, "Save Lake Victoria," was occurring consecutively in six cities across the three countries (Kenya, Uganda,
and Tanzania) that surround the lake in order to highlight the lake's deteriorating quality. As I later learned, this event was not unique; there have
been several periodic calls to save the lake over the years.[20] In attendance
were many NGO representatives, dignitaries including the Mayors of
Kisumu and Homa Bay, and interested public. Additionally, many school-
children were present, several of whom gave presentations involving skits
and songs throughout the afternoon. I noted the event in passing in field
notes, and did not realize its significance until I noticed that the lake played
a background (and sometimes starring) role in many conversations and
local activities over the subsequent weeks and months. The Luo would
sometimes call themselves *Jonam*, or "people of the lake," and the lake was
used for many things. Natural rock formations along some parts of the
lakeshore created convenient places for rows of bathers who used to freely
disrobe and scrub clean in the lake waters. (See figure 17.)

A few meters away, girls would be collecting water to take to their homes to drink and cook; a few meters from them, women would be washing clothes; and a few meters further, grazers would have brought their livestock to drink water from the lake. Further along, one might see some enterprising young men setting up a car wash and using lake water. Many people used to set up small gardens by the lake to grow tomatoes and onions for sale in local markets. Entertaining rowing competitions were held during local festivals for all to enjoy.

Though there were many varied uses of the lake, the most lucrative was fishing. Examining the fishing economy in Nyanza in depth highlights the importance of *place* in shaping HIV outcomes above and beyond individual actions. As illustrated so far, in focusing on the roles of communities, schools, and gendered labor markets in shaping young women's HIV risk, social-structural processes, however global they might be in their reach, are ultimately experienced in local spaces; and features of these local spaces constrain, encourage, and even transform those social structures.[21] Place—both structural (like school) and environmental (like the lake)—is an important characteristic in thinking about sexual networks and the fast spread of disease through them. Denser networks place more people at risk. Denser networks are more likely when all or many of the individuals live in or frequent the same geographic space. Many of the earliest and worst-hit communities in the African AIDS pandemic lived around Lake Victoria. Fishermen and fishing communities and towns were scattered around the lake in Uganda, Tanzania, and Kenya, with migration across water between them and islands in the lake a regular part of everyday life. The lake's geographic centrality to these communities shaped disease transmission and spread in ways I will illustrate. Examining interactions between the ecological environment of Lake Victoria and its surroundings, the gendered fishing economy, and the sexual economy allows us to consider how ecosocial processes might shape HIV outcomes. In this vein, I begin with a discussion of the gendered fishing economy before discussing Lake Victoria and the physical environment around it, both as experienced by the Luo and as discussed in the literature. I then turn to exploring how fisherfolk's sexual relationships and sexual mixing patterns were as much a function of the changing ecological environment in which they fished as they were about the gendered structure of the fishing economy.

## Gendered Transitions into the Fishing Economy

Globally, many fishing economies around the world have gendered structures; that is, men fish and women sell the fish, and this was also the case in Nyanza.[22] Here, fishing was ideally a household affair. Fishermen would fish and then bring their fish back home to their wives who were primarily involved in the fish-handling end of business in a variety of roles. Wives could then sell fish to other women for profit. Women were also involved in drying fish or smoking it on racks by the beach to preserve it (in the absence of refrigeration), buying smoked fish to sell in local and more distant markets, and transporting fish to other parts of the province or country. This gendered division of labor was reflected in the gendered transitions into the fishing industry for young people.

Young boys would start by helping to clean fishing nets, moving on to helping with hauling in fish, eventually becoming a crew member, and slowly accumulating the resources to buy materials to get their boat made and to buy nets and related fishing equipment. (See figure 18.) A typical day for a fisherman, depending on the type of fish he was fishing, would begin with going fishing overnight, spending the morning sleeping, and then spending the afternoon relaxing with friends ahead of another night of fishing. Some also did the *boda boda* business during the day, essentially holding down two physically demanding jobs. There were two levels of fishermen—those who owned their own boats, and thus were responsible for the equipment and for hiring their crew, and those who were crew members. Crew members were not tied to a particular boat and did not have to fish every day. If they wanted to fish, they showed up and were hired at that time. Thus, their income was less secure and was not as great as that of boat owners. While a greater portion of the day's profits went to the boat owner, the remaining portion was evenly distributed among crew members. The boat owner did not always go fishing with his crew (or crews).

As the formal sector declined, and with growing disillusionment with the returns of education, boys and young men in schools near fishing

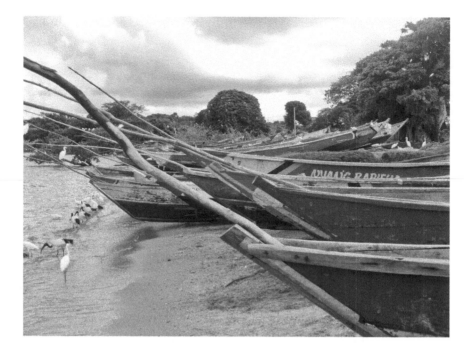

*Figure 18.* Boats by the lake. Photograph by Jackson Wanga.

beaches were especially prone to dropping out. The myriad opportunities to make money at the beach, as well as the clear pathways of upward mobility in the industry, stood in stark contrast to the options they saw for those who stayed in school and graduated but had no employment. Mrs. Oluor, a schoolteacher discussing boys' dropping out of school to fish, explained, "So when a child knows money, that child cannot go to school because they believe that when you go to school you are looking for a future life where you'll be employed and you'll have money. So if at all I can get this money at this particular time, why should I go to school?"[23] The opportunity costs of going to school were very apparent. Every day as they walked home from school, they could see their former classmates, back from fishing, spending their money in local bars and clubs, money that they were not certain school would ultimately bring them.

In addition to these pull factors, there were also push factors for young men. Most of the fishermen I interviewed left school in or at the end of elementary school between the ages of 10 and 16, though a few also left in secondary school. The main reason was lack of school fees since many had dropped out before the government changes. Several said they had to support their parents as well as their own families, while others said that after their parents died, they started fishing to support their siblings. Here is the story of Mark, who, when I asked him how he became a fisherman, described his trajectory:

> With me, I started immediately. I dropped out of school because of the school fees. That was when I was in Form 3 in my second term. . . . Having failed to pay my school fees, I had to come back home and the only solution that could support me was to go to the lake and to start earning a living. That was when I was 18 and immediately I got married. So I had to go and work very hard to support the family. And by then I was very lucky; there was still a lot of fish in the lake and we didn't [need] to buy so many fishing materials. You could even start with very few and at the same time just earn a very good pay.

For Mark, once the possibility of further schooling had ended, he had to find a job to support himself since he could no longer depend on family to support him. His immediate marriage makes sense in light of how the gendered fishing economy here worked—he needed a wife to sell his fish. Also, many fishermen were relatively young, in their 20s or 30s, as his story illustrates, and as many described. This was partly because of high attrition due to the mortality of fishermen even before the time of AIDS. The job of a fisherman involved multiple potentially fatal risks, including encountering hippos or crocodiles (which could kill), attacks by pirates, and drowning. The oldest fisherman I interviewed, Simon, remarked, "What I can say is that I am lucky because I am now 50. If I look behind I don't think that these young gentlemen will sail through up to that age, very few will actually sail up to that age."

For girls and young women, initial forays into the fishing industry were not as independent workers at the beach, but rather as girlfriends and young wives of fishermen. Many of the young women were orphans or were initially schoolgirls going to schools near the beach who thought fishermen were attractive working-class boyfriends. Schoolgirls at a lakeside school noted this in a focus group:

HILLARY:   So in this case you may find a girl only needs money or needs to buy clothes and things she was not having. And other things like the personal effects, like [sanitary] pads. You may see a girl suffering and not even having pads so she will go to the boy for money in order to meet all these needs.

SANYU:   So if a girl wanted to find a guy to help her get money, would that be easy in this community?

HILLARY:   Yes.

ALUOCH:   Fishermen.

PRISCA:   Fishermen.

SANYU:   So is it them looking or the girls looking?

HILLARY:   The girls.

ALUOCH:   All people are hunters.[24]

Along with voluntary transactional relationships with fishermen, female teachers in another setting also discussed relationships not only schoolgirls but also orphans in vulnerable positions had with fishermen in a focus group.

JANET:   You find that maybe both parents of the child have died, and now the child is becoming the breadwinner of the house. There is nothing they can do because the land is there to till but then there is no adequate rain. So nothing happens [i.e., subsistence farming is not possible]. So the [girl]child or boy can decide to go to the beach so that maybe he can help those people fish or maybe sell some fish. Because when you go there automatically you'll come back with money. So when this child goes there, then the child engages herself in activities like immorality, prostitution, something like that. . . . When it is a girl, then they will say *huyo ni wangu* [that one is mine], the men now start fighting over her. And then it continues like that until she will be influenced to live the kind of life that those people are living.

JELINA:   And to add on what she is saying, in fact what she is saying is true because . . . the school which I taught, in fact the teachers were really complaining, the school is near the beach, they were now complaining that they wanted to go the chief and to police because those people at the beach they have money. And now they are cheating the small girls because of that money because they have a lot of money in their hands. Every day they have money. And these schoolgirls or these girls when they see the money, they just go for it. . . . In fact the teacher was telling us that 100 bob [$1] to a kid somewhere down there it's not like money.

MELLIE:  It's not money.

JELINA:  Because she's used to being given even 1000 shillings. Somebody is just giving you for a day.

In the case of orphan girls, many accounts I heard in formal and informal interviews suggested that this situation was often related more to survival, for basic provisions such as food and shelter. Additionally, though, orphan girls who did not feel loved or who felt neglected by their guardians also engaged in relationships with fishermen who they felt provided support that was not just material but also emotional.[25]

In addition to transactional relationships with fishermen, young women also first got involved with fishermen through early marriage to them, often with their parents' blessing. In one community interview among a group of older widows, they noted that girls often married men at the beach in their early teens, with men initiating relationships by wooing girls with presents. In asking why girls married so young, I asked about their parents, and their response suggested that while some parents gave tacit approval, others simply were unaware of how the relationships began:

SANYU:  Where are the parents? Are parents trying to keep them away from men or parents don't mind?

JACINTA:  Parents are negligent. They don't take good care of their daughters. For example if a daughter comes into the house with a present of a petticoat, but the mother sees these presents but she doesn't ask the daughter where she got it from. Maybe the mother is comfortable with it. Then she [the daughter] gets encouraged and goes for money. This way, they get into relationships early with people who give them presents.

Later, another widow said, "The problems are everywhere, even at home. They can even get into the bushes nearby [have sex behind bushes]. Children, especially girls, get into relationships with people like fishermen on the beach because of insufficient money at home. The parents can't afford all their needs, so they have to get into relationships with these men to give them money so that they buy the things that they need. Maybe the parents don't know. It just goes on secretly. The parents cannot know."

As noted earlier, while many young women came from poor households, the gifts and needs were not always for basic survival, and several orphans and nonorphans who engaged in these relationships had parents, guardians, food, and shelter.[26] Fishermen were the quintessential "working-class" men in many communities around Nyanza province. Unlike many who lived on itinerant incomes, fishermen could depend on almost daily money.

In sum, the gendered differences in young people's early engagement with fishing and fishermen reflected the nature of men's and women's roles in the industry. While young men apprenticed their way up, earning independent income from the start, young women's economic dependence on men through transactional and marriage relationships with fishermen was reflected in how they entered and progressed through the fishing industry. Ecological changes wrought significant changes in this gendered and sexual economy in Nyanza with consequences for HIV risk, especially for young women.

## The Significance of Ecology

As I have illustrated in earlier work,[27] the almost 4% annual rate of population growth around the lake, as well as the growth of the fishing industry, had a number of ecological consequences that resulted in significant lake pollution. Sediment runoffs from soil erosion resulting from deforestation (the result of the demand for wood for food preparation and smoking racks for fish), factory waste-dumping, and runoff from fertilizers from nearby farms all contributed to excess nutrients in the lake.[28] These nutrients fueled the fast and disruptive growth of the water hyacinth weed, which covered 6000 hectares of the Kenyan portion of the lake.[29] The weed and pollution in combination had a devastating effect on fish populations in the lake. Not only were the fish breeding grounds destroyed by the weed—reducing both the number and size of fish—but the toxicity of the water drove the surviving fish further out into the lake in search of fresher water. These ecological changes meant both increased competition by fishermen for a now limited number of fish and longer time on the water in search of migrating fish.[30]

Fishermen began spending several days away from home looking for fish, and concerned community members would try to counsel fishermen to return home to their wives more often and not neglect them. The lack of portable refrigeration meant that fishermen needed to land on the nearest beach after a catch to sell their fish before it went bad. However, the rigid and gendered structure of the economy that required a woman to sell fish gave rise to the *jaboya* system.[31] Now, when fishermen landed on a beach far from home, they found a new "wife," with whom they established a sexual relationship, as their primary go-to woman to sell their fish whenever they landed on her beach. *Jaboya* relationships were not considered "commercial" sex relationships since fishermen often established households and had children with the women to whom they gave preferential access to fish.[32] This meant that several fishermen had several homes and families on different beaches. James, a fisherman, noted, "Let's say, like, one who stays [here], suppose he moves from [here] to [another beach], he will be having a family here, and there also he has to have another family."[33] The language of family here further underscores the noncommercial nature of many fishermen's partnerships with fisherwomen. As long as they were at a particular beach, relationships were sustained for a period of time, long enough for intimacy to develop and eventually for a family to be established, but also long enough for HIV transmission and acquisition to occur. However, they were also temporary enough for the HIV viral load to be high enough in the newly infected partner (thus making them highly infectious) to easily spread to the next partner if the fisherman moved on to another beach and the fisherwoman began a relationship with another fisherman. The HIV spread and high partner turnover were also exacerbated by high AIDS-related mortality rates among fishermen, which resulted in several young widows (who had married in their late teens), some of whom were HIV positive, searching for new business and intimate partners. This meant that fishermen, attractive as potential husbands and attractive as rich boyfriends, were also in positions in sexual networks in which they were highly likely to acquire HIV as well as transmit it to their wives and to their partners, who were schoolgirls, young women, and young widows.

The rapid spread of HIV/AIDS throughout the fishing community had started to affect fishermen's attitudes toward relationships. Indeed, during fieldwork, I was conscious of the fact that I was interviewing the fishermen who had survived. They had a firm grasp of HIV/AIDS and how to prevent it; they talked about the many abstinence, monogamy, and condom-use campaigns they had been exposed to, and talked about their experience with voluntary counseling and testing (VCT) to know their HIV status. And while some still knowingly engaged in unprotected sex with concurrent women, they sensed that things were changing and had to change, despite the availability of antiretroviral treatment. As Simon, an older fisherman, reminisced, "when I was starting, ah!, things were so nice, you could have even ten girlfriends but nothing happens. But now, we call it the crocodile, we name it the crocodile, because once you are caught by it, there is no way out, you are dead. Although maybe there is some little hope that we have some certain drugs but physically you are not who you used to be."

The specter of AIDS was changing their attitudes toward multiple relationships, and the meaning of having many girlfriends had changed. Hosea, a younger fisherman, noted, "You know [a long time ago], my parents were telling me, AIDS wasn't there, you were being measured by the number of girlfriends you had, but right now you are being measured by the number of girlfriends you don't have. That's the problem we have right now. Like now, if you have a [large] number of girlfriends, you are as good as dead." The man went on to say that now most of his friends only had one girlfriend. Nonetheless, the damage had already been done, and HIV/AIDS had already decimated many fishermen and members of fishing communities in Nyanza. Further, while many of these men said they were making changes, and despite the widespread knowledge of HIV/AIDS and how to prevent it among fisherfolk, the *jaboya* system still thrives in the fishing industry in Nyanza province.[34]

CONCLUSION

This case study illustrates why young women at home were safer than those who worked. More likely to have recalibrated their needs, those at home were not hostage to the constant need for money and were thus less likely to seek out rich boyfriends in the first place. This meant that they were less likely to meet migrant men positioned in sexual networks of high risk, and that when they found a partner, they were more likely to have bargaining power to demand safe sex or HIV testing before unprotected sex. By contrast, young women in transactional relationships with fishermen boyfriends were having sex with some of the highest-risk partners in this setting, had reduced leverage to demand safe sex from them (because of their high demand as boyfriends), and had a low likelihood of finding a monogamous fisherman boyfriend in this fishing economy.

More broadly, while there are certainly features unique to the fishing economy in Nyanza province, such as the *jaboya* system, gendered economies with highly skewed compensation structures favoring men are a feature of several settings across Africa where HIV prevalence is high. Studies from mining and industrial towns in Southern Africa provide good examples.[35] In several of these settings, men make substantially more money and have more stable jobs; many, because of the long legacy of labor migration, have left their primary wives and girlfriends at home and have transactional or commercial relationships that are temporary with women in the town where they are living. As long as gendered and sexual economies are closely linked, and as long as young women in these settings are powerfully drawn into cultures of consumption, HIV-prevention strategies at the individual level encouraging abstinence, monogamy, and condom use are unlikely to be successful on their own, especially if targeted at the least powerful participants in these economies—young women.

In this setting, young fisherwomen were in a particularly difficult position. The modus operandi in this gendered economy was such that, as long as only men fished and as long as there were limitations on the supply of fish that were driven by the ecology, young women had few or no options out of the sex-for-fish economy. It would be hard for women in this fishing economy who opt out of concurrent sexual relationships with more than one fisherman to get primary and plentiful access to fish. Insisting on a condom may result in no fish that day, since a fisherman would turn to another willing woman. No fisherwoman could depend on the faithfulness of her fisherman partner. Once the fish location had moved, he would land on another beach and find another woman to sell his fish. High fisherman mortality meant that, soon, most women would have to find a new partner anyway.

This case study provides perhaps the clearest example of the limitations of HIV-prevention strategies aimed solely at the individual level, and highlights the essential need to also, in a synergistic fashion, attend to structural and environmental inhibitors constraining the ability of individuals to act to save their own lives.

For residents of Nyanza who regularly made their way to lakeside towns and villages to bury their fisherfolk relatives, their laments, coupled with their visual experience as their *matatu* or *boda boda* passed by the many bars, clubs, and hotels that hosted the vibrant lakeside social life that their deceased loved one no doubt enjoyed, reflected a bitter irony. Those men who were the most financially able to daily exhibit the highly valued good life and who were living along the lake that was so central to life in Nyanza were also those who were dying, and they were taking the young women along with them.

# 7 "To Stem HIV in Africa, Prevent Transmission to Young Women"

A GENDERED AND LIFE-COURSE APPROACH TO HIV PREVENTION

In several African countries where almost half the population is under age 15, millions of girls will be transitioning to adulthood in contexts where prevailing HIV-prevalence rates are 5–10% (in East Africa) and 10–25% (in Southern Africa). The continued existence of these high-HIV-risk environments makes preventing HIV transmission to young women a *critical* goal in order to prevent millions more young women from becoming infected in the years to come. Women in this life-course stage are important to focus on not just in their own right—because of their earlier and higher rates of acquisition of HIV relative to men—but also because of their need for prevention-of-mother-to-child-transmission (PMTCT) programs, as well as because they spend more years on ARV medication compared to men. The large number of young women currently beginning their sexual lives in high HIV-prevalence environments suggest that policy actions (or nonactions) undertaken in the *next five to ten years* may very well determine the course of the HIV pandemic in Africa. In other words, the population of people living with HIV could dramatically increase if everything remains the same. To better focus HIV prevention

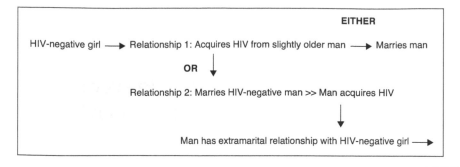

*Figure 19.* The HIV acquisition-transmission cycle.

efforts, it is important to take a life-course perspective in thinking about how HIV is cycling through African populations and therefore how to prevent it.

As previous chapters have illustrated, for this setting and also for other settings in East and Southern Africa, teenage boys have no or relatively low HIV risk. By contrast teenage girls are getting HIV from unmarried men in their early 20s and married men in their 20s and 30s.[1] The primary social drivers of this process of HIV acquisition are relationships with men who are older and slightly older and early marriage, before the age of 20. Girls acquiring HIV before marriage are likely to subsequently pass HIV on to their husbands. As their husbands enter their late 20s and 30s, they then become the older partners of the young unmarried women who have aged into the 15–24 demographic. (See figure 19.)

Disrupting this iterative process is the key to creating, first, an HIV-free cohort of teenage and young women—to match their already HIV-free (or mostly HIV-free) male counterparts—and a subsequent HIV-free cohort of young men and women in their 20s and early 30s. At that point, even if the social dynamics of cross–age group relationships continue, the HIV acquisition-transmission cycle would be broken. Such a disruption would only need to be short term; if maintained for five to ten years, even while HIV may continue to circulate, it would do so at dramatically reduced levels. The implications of this for policy are that HIV interventions for young people should be short, sharp, and effective in order to take full advantage of the window of opportunity provided by the burgeoning population of young women on the verge of their transition through high HIV-prevalence environments. Once the generation of girls currently under 15 has aged into and through high-risk environments, it will be too late, and the numbers of people requiring lifelong antiretroviral therapy will have increased by millions.

## WHAT'S LOVE (AND MONEY) GOT TO DO WITH IT?

The seeming intransigence of individuals' risky behaviors—where they seem to "know but ignore," as I described in chapter 3—reflected not obstinacy or ostrich-like behavior, but rather a rational and interactive response to their social-structural environment. In this book, I have argued that for young women, it was not the fear of getting HIV or AIDS that drove their sexual decision-making. Rather, entanglements of love and money underlay their choices of intimate relationships with the riskiest partners. Further, these relationships occurred and were enabled by key social-structural environments in which their transition to adulthood unfolded—their local communities, their schools, the labor markets they entered, and their ecological environment.

### Individual-Level Interventions

At the individual level, for young women, relationship transitions were intertwined with their transformation into "consuming women" who want to become beautiful and desirable women in the face of their own economic limitations. This made young women financially dependent on the men they partnered with if they wanted to become ideal Luo women and find love with a providing man. Regular condom use in such longer-term relationships was difficult. Young men, unable to afford sustaining, long-term "relationships for sex" were often involuntarily abstinent or had relationships with nonconsuming women, thus avoiding HIV risk. In this way, the social mechanisms for the maintenance of low HIV rates among young men were already in place. The pursuit of education for young women involved pursuing transactional relationships to meet "new" and continual modern gendered needs for things such as sanitary pads, toiletries, and cosmetics that arose as they pursued education. Finding a job involved long periods of waiting and uncertainty, and exacerbated need after there had already been a reduction of financial support from parents and guardians. This meant that to supplement meager wages from "small small" jobs, they engaged in relationships with working men with money, and, particularly in Nyanza, with fishermen whose sexual lifestyles were risky, in order to meet their needs.

What was putting young women at risk in this context, then, was not so much the fact that they engaged in sex, but rather with whom they engaged in sex. In other words, it was *the logic of partner choice*—preferring older or slightly older providing boyfriends and ignoring same-age poor boyfriends—that placed them at risk. One way to counter this logic in the face of their widespread knowledge about abstinence, being faithful, and condom use (ABC) would be to provide different kinds of knowledge—in particular, as Pascaline Dupas has argued, specifically showing girls their high likelihood of getting HIV from partners who are a different age. In this context, teenage women's risk is from young men in their 20s and 30s. Because of this, the most critical information goal, now that basic information is widespread, is telling them that. In other words, a simple presentation and explanation of figure 11 in chapter 4 might be enough to encourage young women to seek their same-aged counterparts as partners. Dupas demonstrated that when the teenage girls in her study in Western Kenya were told about the dangers of cross-generational relationships, a follow-up a year later showed a 28% decline in pregnancies. Most of the reduction was in relationships with older partners. Meanwhile, girls reported an increase in sexual partnerships with young men their age; however, there was no increase in teenage-partner pregnancies, suggesting that they were increasing condom use with same-aged partners, with whom they presumably had more bargaining power. She argues that it was more effective to encourage girls to shift from risky (older partner, unprotected) sex to safer sex (in regard to HIV) than to tell them not to have sex at all. This approach respects young women's agency, and allows them to do their own cost-benefit analysis about which relationships to choose, and to weigh their consumption needs and desires against the risk of getting HIV. This then gives young women incentives to shift their logic of partner choice. Along with this new knowledge, leveraging women's agency in the entering and exiting of relationships may also be useful. Specifically, if young women still want to choose older partners, knowing the HIV-prevalence environment and the particular risk these partners might pose may increase their incentive to insist on HIV testing before beginning sex. Testing at the beginning of the relationship is important, as the agency may be lost once the relationship and provision has begun.

Among young men, while, as noted earlier, the social mechanisms for low HIV risk are already in place, educating them while they are a captive audience in school will be critical in enabling them to stay HIV free as they age. Schoolboys should also be taught about their HIV-risk environment, and particularly how their HIV rates climb as they age. This knowledge should be coupled with practical sessions on how to use a condom, the importance of HIV testing before abandoning condom use, and the importance of practicing "zero grazing"—reducing the numbers of partners they have, even when they finally have the money at older ages to afford concurrent partners. Finally, it may also be useful to educate boys and young men about the benefits of male circumcision, which, as described in chapter 1, has been shown to significantly reduce the risk of HIV acquisition.[2]

Community workshops with similar information for young men and women out of school, and for middle-aged men, may also be usefully held. Educating men is an important part of creating and preserving a HIV-free cohort of young people.

### Institutional-Level Interventions

Young women's social-structural *environments* also enabled and facilitated their partner choices. They pursued beauty—the modern way—in response to changing sociocultural ideals of what constituted a beautiful woman. Further, the entanglement of relationship transitions with cultural ideals of beauty and the explicit globalized cultivation of desire for things requiring continual consumption occurred in a gendered economic context where men had greater access to income than women. Thus, providing older men with access to regular income were partners who enabled young women to meet these ideals, even while they waited for men closer to their own age to accumulate the income to eventually support a consuming wife. Money was not only central to the initiation and maintenance of relationships, but also crucial in paving the path for those relationships to transition into marriage, an institution that, in this setting, also determined HIV chances.

School, an institution that embodied modernity, contributed to the production of young women as modern consuming women. The pursuit of education brought large numbers of girls into a structural context where peer groups constructed gendered norms about what products counted as necessities and facilitated normative environments in which relationships with providing men were acceptable and desirable. Further, young women were in close daily contact with men in the age and economic group of risk—older male teachers with regular access to income. In an ambiguous and contradictory cultural context where transactional sex was both condemned and admired, and in which teachers, as one of the few salaried groups in a small community, were highly valued, relationships between teachers and students were not as highly sanctioned as they should have been. A renewed effort to sanction deviant teachers would be essential to end this structural vulnerability.

Additionally, given the widespread mention of sanitary towels as the most regular need among schoolgirls, the provision of menstrual solutions should be routinized in schools with girls. In schools that have water availability, a routinized shift to the use of menstrual cups, which are eco-friendly, washable, and recyclable, and are low-cost devices requiring a one-time cost of about $25 each, may be a viable option. This cost (what schoolgirls would spend in one to two years on pads) can no doubt be significantly reduced if produced on a mass scale.[3] If they are introduced to girls as "modern" devices and used by every female student, this would not only ensure that users were not being stigmatized, but also remove monthly dependencies on money to buy pads. Further, even girls who dropped out of school could continue to use them.

A series of studies in Africa is beginning to investigate the use of conditional cash transfers to schoolgirls for HIV prevention. For example, a study in Malawi was conducted and recently described by Sarah Baird and colleagues in a series of papers.[4] They found that families and their girls in school who were given subsidies ($4 to the household, $1 pocket money to the girl) reported less frequent sex, were less likely to have a partner over the age of 25, and had lower adjusted odds of being HIV or HSV-2 positive. The findings suggest that when girls were given pocket money and enabled to stay in school because of school fee provision, they did not choose older partners. In a similar fashion to Dupas discussed earlier, a combination of HIV-prevalence information and small financial provision jointly reduced the attractiveness of the riskiest partners for young women's HIV acquisition.

As noted in chapter 5, large majorities of girls do not complete high school. Focusing on this demographic of women—those out of school up to 24 years old—is particularly critical, especially since this is the crucial period when they transition into marriage, a relationship in which perhaps their greatest risk for HIV acquisition exists. Thus, creating structural environments that enable them to enter marriage HIV-free or at least marry a partner whose HIV status they know is important. The same Malawi research by Sarah Baird and colleagues on unconditional cash transfers to girls who drop out of school and the households they lived in suggests that continuing to support these girls may yield benefits in terms of delayed marriage and reduced pregnancies. This is important in trying to prevent early marriage (before age 20). Girls who do not *have to* get married at this stage, especially since the household is being subsidized and is not necessarily in a hurry to get bride wealth from a daughter's husband-to-be, are more likely to be in a better bargaining position for safe sex and HIV testing of partners before marriage.

Conditional cash transfer programs may be a particularly useful part of a short-term strategy to create an HIV-free cohort of young people. However, policy planners should think through and thoroughly investigate potential resistance and backlash in communities that may result from, for example, giving pocket money to girls and not boys (the latter of whom are often ignored or simply overlooked in development interventions).

The pursuit of employment as youth transitioned out of school led them to face a gendered job market—gendered in such a way that the types of jobs to which women, in contrast to young men, had access to were "small small" jobs, which, for young women, brought little income, insufficient to meet their greater perceived needs. Young women's relationships with some of these men who worked—fishermen—connected them to a network structure of high HIV risk characterized by high rates of concurrency. This concurrency, in turn, was enabled by changing ecological environments shaping fishermen's behavior. HIV prevalence is high in settings where gendered access to income and jobs is highly skewed, with men earning many times more money than women. To the extent possible, opening up *all* job opportunities to women is the best way to start dismantling the connection between gendered and sexual economies. In Nyanza, the best innovation would be to enable young women to also fish. Initially, this would require training young and middle-aged women in how to set up their boats and fishing equipment, and how to fish. Subsequently, they can apprentice younger women going forward. Teaching women how to fish will completely remove men's leverage of sex in the sex-for-fish economy. Women can simply buy and sell from other women and have access to their own daily money.[5] Aside from encouraging the creation of new businesses, this intervention recognizes that a lot can be done to level compensation structures *within* existing industries.

The recognition of the connections between economic need, gendered inequality in access to income, and HIV acquisition has led to increasing interest in the use of microfinance programs for HIV interventions.[6] However, so far, programs that have aimed to provide *young* women with microcredit to start their own businesses have met with limited success. In Kenya, the TRY Program, working with young women living in informal settlements in Nairobi, gave them microcredit but found that the program foundered with very low rates of repayment, the disappearance of participants, and sometimes the co-optation of the money for other uses. The program found that without close mentorship, commitment by loan officers living in the same community as the women, and focused follow-up—a highly labor-intensive and thus rare process—these programs would not work.[7]

SHAZ!, a program conducted in Zimbabwe among 16–19-year-old orphans who were out of school, found similar challenges. The project combined life-skills and HIV training with business training and microloan provision. Repayment after six months in the program was very low—only 20% had begun repayment and only 6% had repaid in full. Thus, over 70% had not paid anything. Young women encountered a lot of challenges in starting their businesses, including theft and confiscation of their goods, having to bribe police, threats to their personal safety, lack of a place to store their money, and theft of their money. Additionally, lack of trust of their mentors and lack of money to attend regular meetings also hindered their progress. Girls with family support were the most successful in the program. Overall, however, many young women were at *greater* risk for HIV as a result of their increased vulnerability once they had begun the program.[8]

The most successful program to date is IMAGE, which was carried out in South Africa. The program enrolled young and middle-aged women up to the age of 49. The program gave microloans to women and also combined gender and HIV training into the regular meetings. When focusing on results from the youngest recipients of microloans in the program (aged 14–35, with an average age of 29), they found that young women were more likely to have gone for HIV testing and less likely to have had unprotected sex with a nonspouse.[9] This suggests that having their own money and business gave them more bargaining power in relationships to demand safe sex and testing. Additionally, involvement in a program with middle-aged women helped provide additional community support for the young women that was lacking in the SHAZ! and TRY programs. Having inbuilt and on-the-ground mentorship from women in the community whom they knew and who are accountable for things other than the business was likely part of the program's success.

In addition to the downsides of microfinance documented earlier (high default rates, co-optation of money for other uses, and the potential increased vulnerability of young women to HIV) microfinance programs have also been criticized more broadly for what they often represent— women's inability to find well-paid work. The growing provision of microfinance to women in developing countries, scholars argue, masks the retreat of the state from the provision of services, with women's unpaid labor and nongovernmental organizations often picking up the slack. The state retreat is explicitly linked to globalization and global institutions that pushed structural-adjustment programs that pressured governments to reduce public spending, open up markets, and provide incentives (such as lower labor restrictions) to encourage foreign direct investment. For many African countries, structural-adjustment policies have not worked, and while microfinance programs benefit some women as they start up small businesses that eventually become successful, many others remain entrenched in the unstable informal sector, or become more deeply entrenched in debt and poverty.[10]

A key way forward that emerges from these critiques is to revision microfinance programs as part of a larger strategy in the country to develop local communities as a whole. In 2009, for example, the Kenyan government launched a program called Kazi Kwa Vijana. The program, meaning literally "work for youth," combines job opportunities in public-works programs and provides income-generating funds to young men and women for community projects to start businesses. While the program has had its challenges, it provides one example of state-led development that provides employment for young people.[11] The new constitution in Kenya redesigned the country's governance by devolving power to counties. The hope of this strategy is, at least in part, that it will support development and self-governance at the community level. Linking microfinance programs to community-development plans is one way to combine increasing the opportunities for young women and increasing the availability of more stable jobs, while helping communities move out of poverty. One possible way this could look would be to create women-led village and town-level committees within each county to identify community needs, encourage multigenerational (youth and middle-aged) group proposals of businesses to meet those needs, create a budget for a community-businesses fund from county budgets (with potential private partnerships with local community members and businesses that can also provide training), and create a system to provide start-up grants or low-interest loans to fund a portion of these businesses. The community nature of these proposals and businesses would help reduce some of the pitfalls of programs noted earlier: it would potentially reduce default rates, reduce the possibility of co-optation of money for other uses, and have community and county buy-in to enable them to succeed.

Finally, as noted in chapter 1, the natural environment is an oft-ignored actor in HIV prevention, yet it is a critical piece of not just many local and national economies, but also people's everyday lives. Paying attention to the ecosocial environment and its interactions with labor markets is critical. In this setting, environmental changes to the lake and population ecology enabled and fueled the *jaboya* sex-for-fish system. Trying to encourage fisherwomen to use condoms, without understanding their ecostructural limitations, would be an exercise in futility.[12] Creating a stable ecosystem—with fresh water for fish to live and breed in—would create a structural environment in which fishermen could engage in "zero-grazing," reducing the number of families they started, reducing the necessary scope of their travels, and limiting the number of beaches on which they landed. An abundance of fish in the lake and women fishers to buy fish from would make it much easier for fisherwomen to insist on safe sex and HIV testing in any relationships they have.

## NOT JUST NYANZA

While many elements of this reality and these policy suggestions are unique to Luo-Nyanza, I have shown throughout the book that the gendered social-structural processes evidenced in this setting express themselves across the continent. Indeed, in seeing the extent to which the experience of the Luo community contributes to understanding the gendered disparity in HIV rates in other parts of the continent, there appear many similarities. While the love of the good life—*raha*—had a particular iteration in the Luo community, this yearning is evident in many African communities where modern commodities such as mobile phones, fashionable clothing, and other such goods are prized. Youth in many parts of West, Central, East, and Southern Africa desire and seek the good life through the consumption of modern products yet, like Luo-Nyanza youth, lack the financial means to attain them.[13] As documented in chapter 2, throughout the continent, pursuing relationships with providing men as a means for enhanced consumption has become a normalized and common strategy for young African women. Additionally, having providing partners has become a major mechanism, outside of marriage, through which the gendered and generational redistribution of money and resources is occurring. These similarities across settings mean that the policy interventions suggested here may have applicability beyond Nyanza province. In other words, changing the content of HIV education to include information about the specific HIV-risk environment young people are navigating, keeping school safe for girls, increasing job access for young women, ensuring gender equity in pay among young people, and paying attention to the ecosocial interactions and the natural environment will be important in several African settings.

The historical antecedents for these connections between gendered and sexual economies push us to question the extent to which young women's higher HIV risk is so extraordinary. Is HIV/AIDS merely highlighting, albeit in a deadly fashion, persisting social structures that through different incarnations have always positioned young women in categories of high risk? In this instance, I argue that this is not the case. There are many motivations for transactional sex such as independence and emotional, sexual, and social freedom, but what is different is the historical shift in both the value and the uses of money among young African women, a shift toward ever-increasing consumption, and the desire for things that require continual replenishing and thus continual transacting. The continual nature of these desires moves young women's needs beyond the ability of what most families can afford, and without economic infrastructures that generate well-paying jobs for young women, consuming women will continue to be dependent on providing men to become modern.

The tragic epidemiological consequences of this shift are the continual motivation for young women to sustain the riskiest partnerships (longer-term relationships with men who are in the highest age group of risk) and a motivation to simultaneously curtail or postpone the safest partnerships (relationships with men their own age). It is critical to move beyond the immediate questions about sexual behavior (such as why women are not using condoms and why men are having multiple relationships) and immediate solutions (such as teaching girls how to negotiate safe sex and telling men to be faithful, and so on). Instead, they should be *accompanied* in each context by approaches that unpack the logics of partner choice, particularly around the relationships, their emotional content (for example, love) and money, the connections between the gendered and sexual economy in a particular community and school setting, and the role of the ecological environment. This knowledge would enable useful combinations of individual-level and structural solutions that would reduce young women's HIV risk across the continent.

The current crossroads presents an extraordinary window of opportunity: to bring the HIV epidemic to a halt by maintaining HIV-free cohorts of young people or to allow a dramatic increase in the numbers of young women living with HIV when they are exposed to prevailing HIV risk environments. It is hoped that this book not only provides a new impetus to this important and urgent conversation, but also encourages a focused and concerted effort immediately and over the next few years, as the next generation of young people transition to adulthood, to begin an end to the HIV/AIDS pandemic.

# Epilogue  The Magic Bullet?

The statistics from the latest UNAIDS report, while still grim, suggest that the tide is turning on the HIV/AIDS pandemic in sub-Saharan Africa.[1] The estimated number of new cases remains high at 1.8 million each year, but that is 25% lower than 2001, which saw 2.4 million new cases. The subcontinent still accounts for 71% of new infections globally, but it has seen the second-largest decline (25%) across world regions. Additionally, life-prolonging antiretroviral therapy (ART) is starting to be rolled out across the continent. Currently just over half (56%) of Africans who need the medication are receiving it.[2] Reflecting this progress, while the subcontinent continues to annually account for 70% (1.2 million) of AIDS deaths, there has been a 32% decline in AIDS-related mortality. Because of this, fewer children are becoming orphaned, fewer people are losing their spouses and partners, and fewer families are losing their primary breadwinners. This is hopeful news. However, the nature of AIDS in the absence of a cure is such that progress in the next few years will be represented by a stable or *growing* number of people living with HIV. The number of people living with HIV/AIDS (PLWHA) in Africa has increased to 23.5 million (up from 20.9 million people in 2001). Indeed, even if HIV-prevalence rates remain stable, we can still expect to see millions more PLWHA. (A declining number of PLWHA would mean that increasing numbers of people are dying of the disease.) Many of these millions will be young women. The continued growth of PLWHA is particularly challenging in light of what is currently the biggest intervention to keep them alive: ART/ARV drugs. This is medication that these millions of Africans, and young women in particular (as they acquire HIV earlier and at higher rates) will need for the rest of their lives.

ARV drugs have a dramatic and swift "Lazarus effect" on people with advanced HIV or AIDS. By suppressing HIV, which would otherwise destroy the immune system, the progression of the disease from HIV to AIDS is slowed and even reversed, enabling people to live for 20 or more years with the virus. People who are wasting away in their beds gain weight and energy and, within a few weeks or months, are able to resume their regular active lives. Remarkable developments in the last decade, and the last three years in particular, have demonstrated that ARV drugs are effective not only at prolonging the lives of people living with HIV, but also for preventing the onward transmission of the virus to others by reducing the amount of the virus (the viral load) in an HIV-positive person's system.[3] The promise of ARVs—not just for prolonging lives, but for limiting onward transmission—has led to its increasingly being perceived as the magic bullet in the fight against HIV/AIDS.

## ART as Prevention

In Africa, limited resources mean that ART is given to the sickest PLWHA—those with very low white-blood-cell counts. The problem with this approach from an HIV-prevention standpoint is that viral load (and thus infectiousness) is highest at two points: in the first year of HIV acquisition, when most people are asymptomatic, the disease is invisible, and they are probably ignorant of their status, and again six to ten years later, when they start to transition to AIDS and are symptomatic and regularly sick. By the time someone gets on ARV medication, they have already had about six years of potential transmission to their sexual partners.[4] For prevention purposes, it makes sense to give ARVs early, as a number of studies that I will briefly discuss have recently demonstrated.

Substantial HIV transmission in sub-Saharan Africa happens between stable heterosexual couples. That is, like Mara and her partner in chapter 4, a large number of couples are sero-discordant, where one member is HIV positive and one is HIV negative. A person who is part of a sero-discordant couple not only is more likely to get HIV from their partner (as opposed to through an extramarital relationship), but also has about a 10% annual risk of acquisition.[5] Because of the predominance of women infected with HIV in Africa, there is now little to no gender difference in who the HIV-positive partner (the index partner) is in sero-discordant partnerships.[6] The most prominent study examining ART as prevention was among such couples. In a study conducted among 1763 sero-discordant couples in nine African countries by Myron Cohen and colleagues, there was a 96% relative reduction in HIV transmission when the HIV-positive partner was given ARV drugs early.[7] This study demonstrated that early "test and treat" programs could be remarkably effective in HIV prevention. Jared Baeten and colleagues, following 4758 couples in Kenya and Uganda, sought to examine whether giving ARV drugs to the HIV-*negative* partner would reduce their likelihood of acquiring HIV (preexposure prophylaxis). They found a 75% reduction in HIV incidence among negative partners given the once-a-day Truvada drug; among those with high adherence to the drug, they found an 82% reduction in HIV incidence.[8]

The critical challenge with ARV medication, which was highlighted in these studies, is drug adherence, taking the drug as regularly as prescribed.[9] Drug adherence to HIV medication is critical not just for the preventive purposes described above, but also because a lapse can result in rapid development of drug-resistant HIV in a patient, making them unable to use the drug again. Drug adherence was a key factor differentiating effective interventions in the studies of couples and ineffective interventions in studies among young women. The most prominent of these—FEM-PREP—was conducted in Kenya, South Africa, and Tanzania by Lut Van Damme and colleagues among 2120 young women aged 18–35, a third of whom were married. They found no significant difference in HIV incidence between participants on treatment and those not on treatment. Less than 40% of the respondents were adherent to the drug partly, the authors hypothesize, because they did not perceive themselves to be at risk.[10] This suggests that ART as prevention might not be as helpful as a prevention strategy among young women, who are at disproportionate risk of acquiring HIV, and who may, with low adherence, develop drug resistance to some ART should they ever need it.

### ARV Drugs and Economic Sustainability

There has also been a substantial debate about whether the ART scale-up in Africa is going to be financially sustainable. ARV drugs are extraordinarily expensive. Global pharmaceutical companies were vilified for many years after drugs to delay the transition from HIV to AIDS were first discovered and delivered. The primary reason for this was the high cost of medications, sometimes as high as $1,000 a month, accessible to people in the West with health insurance or governments that subsidized or covered those drugs, as well as to the very wealthy in Africa.[11] With these costs, the vast majority of people who needed the medication could not afford it and were dying by the millions. This was increasingly and widely perceived by the global public as ethically unacceptable.

The economic rationale for high drug prices from the point of view of the pharmaceutical companies was straightforward. The cost of bringing a drug to market (from invention to production) has been estimated at $4 to $12 billion dollars spent over a period of between eight to 12 years. While patents are available for 20 years, they are usually filed while drug trials are ongoing. Trials can take up to 10 years before they are ready for widespread dissemination. By the time a drug comes to market, there may only be eight to 10 years left on the patent. A drug like Viread used by 8/10 newly diagnosed patients in the United States brings in annual profits of about $2 billion a year. This means that drug companies only have two to six years to recoup their $4 to $12 billion dollars of research and development costs before they start to realize a profit.[12] In a battle now well documented, after several years of global activism on several continents, legal battles, and competition in the form of generic drug production from companies in India and China, Western pharmaceutical companies finally bowed to pressure and reduced their prices, first for mother-to-child transmission drugs and then for adult drugs.[13] Gilead, the parent company of Viread, for example, decided to engage in no profit provision of the drug to 68 developing countries. This meant a 30-day supply of drugs at $24.71 or $0.82

per day, which reflected the cost of manufacturing and administering the drug.[14] The medication has thus become, seemingly, very affordable. However, even at a cost of about a dollar or so a day, the millions of people across the continent requiring the drug daily for the rest of their lives—for young women this would be at least 30–40 years—still make it economically unsustainable for poor countries, this side of a cure.[15] (I describe and estimate the costs of a hypothetical early "test and treat" program for young women in endnote 15 and table A5 in the appendix.) This is one reason why ARVs are given to the sickest and closest to death rather than those who are still healthy. While many African countries, notably South Africa, have significantly increased their domestic investment in HIV prevention and treatment, at least 26 African countries rely for 50%–75% of their AIDS budget on international donors such as the United States and its PEPFAR program.[16] For many poor countries, HIV is by no means the most important issue. Widespread poverty and the associated challenges such as clean water, more immediate health problems other than HIV resulting in high infant mortality, and trying to expand education and improve local infrastructure present more immediate problems. And how long can Africans depend on international donors to keep paying for the drugs?

The biggest argument for its use, however, is that the reduction of HIV incidence in the short term will result in long-term payoffs in reduced morbidity and thus reduced need for medications as well as reduced mortality. Early testing and treatment, the argument goes, will eventually pay for itself.[17] Even if this is true, the amount of money involved, potentially billions of dollars, provides an impetus to think hard about cheaper and short-term solutions that are still effective for HIV prevention in order to limit the number of people who are eventually going to need ARVs. Low-cost prevention is 28 times more cost effective than ARV treatment, especially when measuring the cost of condom use versus the cost of lifetime ARV treatment.[18] Efforts to scale up ART across sub-Saharan Africa and ensure that everyone who needs the medication can get it are critical and important. However, they should not shift focus from the need for basic HIV prevention that does not require medication. That is, engaging in HIV prevention that does not involve millions of young women having to be on ART—for prevention of HIV acquisition or transmission—for the rest of their lives.

## THE SOCIAL VACCINE

If history is to be believed, it is unlikely that HIV biomedicine alone will ultimately be responsible for dramatic declines in HIV incidence. The epidemiological transition in the United States in the twentieth century—the shift from predominantly infectious-disease causes of death (for example, polio and measles) to chronic-disease causes of death (for example, cancer and heart disease)—is popularly thought to be the result of biomedical interventions. However, as John and Sonja McKinlay demonstrated in confirmation of the McKeown hypothesis, mortality due to a variety of common infectious diseases, including measles, scarlet fever, tuberculosis, typhoid, pneumonia, influenza, whooping cough, diphtheria, and poliomyelitis, substantially declined *well before* vaccines and medication came on the scene. It was public health campaigns such as improving public sanitation, increasing hygiene in hospitals, and improved nutrition that played a large role. Vaccines and cures were more significant in preventing the reemergence of new epidemics and maintaining low levels of the disease in the population than they were in bringing down existing epidemics.[19] If history repeats itself with the HIV/AIDS pandemic, other sorts of interventions may contribute to a dramatic decline in HIV incidence before a cure appears.

Indeed, the few African countries that have seen significant declines in their HIV epidemic did not achieve this with biomedicine, but with sociostructurally engineered, supported, and enabled individual changes in behavior that eventually had population-wide impact. While there continues to be skepticism in the AIDS research community about behavior change, in Uganda there is now scientific consensus that delayed age at first sex among youth, casual and commercial sex-partner reduction ("zerograzing"), and, to a lesser degree, increased condom use among nonspousal partners—in that order—were the critical changes that resulted in a dramatic decline in HIV incidence.[20] In other words, "abstinence—be faithful—condom use" was locally operationalized as "delay, reduce, and if necessary, condomize." Critically, these actions were not promoted in isolation. Indeed, the level of strategic and concerted action was extraordinary. Uganda's president, Yoweri Museveni, personally involved himself in AIDS-awareness education as he traveled around the country. As Green and colleagues document, in addition to this high-level political support, involvement by multiple sectors of government and civil society (secular and faith-based) and an aggressive public media campaign that was decentralized and community-based contributed to an enabling structural environment for individual actions that led to an HIV epidemic decline. The indigenous nature of this effort was reflected by the relatively low cost to donors—$180 million between 1989 and 1998.[21] In the historical vein discussed earlier, the key role of the now widespread availability of ARV drugs in Uganda is, arguably, not just keeping many people alive who would have otherwise died, but also maintaining relatively low HIV incidence levels by keeping community viral loads down and thereby reducing the chance of onward transmission. (While there has been a slight increase in the HIV prevalence in the country since its decline, it has not returned to the highs of the 1980s or 1990s.) In this way, biomedicine played a critical but not primary role in the sequence of long-term HIV prevention.

Adding a social-structural layer to individual-level interventions reflects a recognition that individuals do not operate in social vacuums, but rather make decisions in environments that enable or disable particular kinds of actions. Changing gendered, economic, ecological, normative, and organizational structural contexts can help individuals make choices that enable their long-term health and well-being.[22] This is particularly important since a focus on strategies aimed at individual young women will be useless as long as there are structural mechanisms in place that keep reproducing the same gendered and generational structural environments that have produced their disproportionate risk in the first place. ARV drugs are an important part of the fight against HIV/AIDS. However, they must be combined with multilevel social vaccines to end young women's HIV risk and begin an end to te HIV/AIDS pandemic in Africa.

# Appendix

| Table A1 | Mortality Rates (per 1000) for Children under Five in Nyanza Province and Kenya, 1979–2009 | |
|---|---|---|
| Year | Nyanza province | Kenya |
| 1979–1989 | 148.5 | 90.9 |
| 1993 | 186.8 | 93.2 |
| 1998 | 198.8 | 105.2 |
| 2003 | 206 | 115 |
| 2008–2009 | 149 | 74 |

Data from KDHS 1989, 1994, 1999, 2004, and 2010.

*Table A2*     2010 HIV Prevalence Rates of Young Luo-Nyanza
Women and Men, by Age Group with 95%
Confidence Intervals (in Parentheses) and Sample
Sizes (N)

| Age Group | Women (%) | Men (%) |
|---|---|---|
| 15–19 | **15.66 (7.37–23.96)** | **2.74 (0–6.31)** |
| 20–24 | 17.43 (9.38–25.46) | 8.49 (0–17.46) |
| 25–29 | 34.21 (20.26–48.16) | 28.70 (13.08–44.33) |
| 30–34 | 31.25 (13.58–48.93) | 29.36 (10.13–48.59) |
| Total | 22.26 (16.8–27.7) | 12.53 (7.48–17.58) |
| (N) | N = 292 | N = 234 |

DATA: KDHS 2010.

*Table A3*     2004 HIV Prevalence Rates of Young Luo-Nyanza
Women and Men, by Age Group with 95%
Confidence Intervals (in Parentheses) and Sample
Sizes (N)

| Age group | Women (%) | Men (%) |
|---|---|---|
| 15–19 | **5.7 (0.5–10.9)** | **0 (no observations)** |
| 20–24 | **45.1 (29.7–60.5)** | **10.6 (0.4–21.6)** |
| 25–29 | 29.2 (11.7–46.7) | 45.5 (21.7–69.2) |
| 30–34 | 27.0 (10.8–43.2) | 30.5 (6.8–54.2) |
| Total | 24.5 (17.6–31.4) | 13.4 (7.3–19.3) |
| (N) | N = 185 | N = 136 |

DATA: KDHS 2004.

*Table A4*    HIV Prevalence by Currently Working Status, by Age Group, with 95% Confidence Intervals (in Parentheses) and Sample Sizes

| Age group | Kenyan women (N = 2227) | | Luo-Nyanza women (N = 254) | |
|---|---|---|---|---|
| | NO PAID WORK | PAID WORK | NO PAID WORK | PAID WORK |
| 15–29 | **4.1 (2.8–5.5)** | **9.0 (6.5–11.6)** | **13.1 (7.0–19.2)** | **29.2 (19.7–38.7)** |
| 15–19 | 2.1 (0.9–3.3) | 4.6 (0.9–8.2) | 13.2 (4.1–22.3) | 21.7 (3.4–40.0) |
| 20–24 | 4.1 (1.5–6.7) | 8.8 (5.2–12.5) | 9.1 (1.9–16.4) | 26.6 (12.4–40.9) |
| 25–29 | 9.4 (4.5–14.2) | 10.8 (6.4–15.3) | 25.3 (2.7–50.3) | 35.9 (18.7–53.2) |

*Table A5*    Estimated Annual Cost to Provide ARV Medication to HIV-Positive Young Women

| Country | HIV prevalence (%) among young women, by age group | | Midyear total population size (2012) | Number of HIV-positive women, 15–24 years old | Annual cost at $1 a day |
|---|---|---|---|---|---|
| | 15–19 | 20–24 | | | |
| Kenya | 2.7 | 6.4 | 4,300,000 | 391,300 | $142,824,500 |
| Malawi | 4.2 | 6.4 | 1,590,000 | 168,540 | $61,517,100 |
| South Africa | 6.7 | 21.1 | 5,110,000 | 1,420,580 | $518,511,700 |
| Uganda | 3.0 | 7.1 | 3,560,000 | 359,560 | $131,239,400 |
| Zambia | 5.7 | 11.8 | 1,370,000 | 239,750 | $87,508,750 |
| Zimbabwe | 4.2 | 10.6 | 1,260,000 | 186,480 | $68,065,200 |
| Total | | | | | $1,009,666,650 |

NOTES: HIV prevalence rates (KDHS 2010; MDHS 2010; Rehle et al. 2010; Uganda AIS 2012; ZDHS 2007; ZHDS 2010–11). The mid-2012 population is based on population pyramids from DHS where the average population size of 15–19 and 20–24 year olds ranges between 4.5% and 5% in each of these countries. I have thus assumed that all 15–24 year olds combined compose about 10% of the populations of the countries. I then calculated their population size using mid-2012 projections from the Population Reference Bureau (2012) world data sheet. **For the number of those HIV positive:** I applied the HIV-prevalence rates from DHS for young women in these age groups to the population size to derive an estimate of the number of young women who are HIV positive in each country. **For the cost of ARVs,** I multiplied the number of those who are HIV positive by 365 to derive an annual estimated cost of ARVs if ARVs cost $1 a day.

# Notes

## 1. A STUBBORN DISPARITY

1. Glynn et al. 2001.

2. UNAIDS 2012.

3. UNAIDS 2009.

4. "HIV prevalence" refers to the percentage of a particular population who are infected, in this case 15–19-year-old girls. Laga et al. 2001:931.

5. Population Reference Bureau 2012.

6. That is, even if HIV-prevalence levels remain the same, the absolute number of victims will increase because of growing populations.

7. In sub-Saharan African countries where nationally representative Demographic and Health Surveys (DHS) or AIDS Indicator Surveys (AIS) HIV-prevalence data were available, including for Swaziland (2006–7), Uganda (2004–5), Rwanda (2005), Lesotho (2004), Ethiopia (2005), Guinea (2005), Burkina Faso (2003), Cameroon (2004), Cote d'Ivoire (2005), Ghana (2003), Liberia (2007), and Senegal (2005), almost all show similar gendered disparities between 15–24-year-old youth, with young women across these age groups having higher HIV-prevalence levels than same-aged young men. There were four exceptions: in the Democratic Republic of Congo (2007) and Mali (2006) surveys, 15–19-year-old men had higher HIV-prevalence rates than same-aged women (but this later reversed, with 20–24-year old women having slightly higher rates than young men); in the Tanzania AIS (2003–4) and Niger survey,

15-19-year-old men and women had a similar prevalence level, but 20-24-year-old women had higher prevalence levels (ORC Macro Intl.). See also Gouws et al. 2008.

8. UNAIDS 2012.

9. Life expectancy with HIV in the absence of medication is about six to ten years. See graphs in Gouws et al. 2008.

10. See Hogan and Astone 1986; Shanahan 2000; Furstenberg 2000; Lloyd 2005 for the transition-to-adulthood framework; see Ruddick 2003 for the Western peculiarity of the model; and see Mensch, Bruce, and Greene 1998; Lloyd, Kaufman, and Hewett 2000; and Lloyd 2005 for applications to the African context.

11. See Rindfuss 1991 for his discussion of demographic density of the life course among young people; see also Mojola 2011b.

12. Ruddick 2003; Johnson-Hanks 2002, 2006.

13. Comaroff and Comaroff 2000; Cole and Durham 2007.

14. Abimiku and Gallo 1995; Bolan, Ehrhardt, and Wasserheit 1999; Zabin and Kiragu 1998; Gupta and Mahy 2003; Bouvet et al. 1989; Glynn et al. 2001; see also Higgins, Hoffman, and Dworkin 2010.

15. Royce et al. (1997) estimate that 15%–25% of HIV transmission might be accounted for by nonsexual forms of transmission such as blood transfusion and infected needles. Young African women's greater and repeated exposure to health care systems, compared to young men, may be a particular avenue of risk, in their going for prenatal care requiring blood tests, in their hospitalization for giving birth, and in the case of pregnancy complications, as well as in their role as medical staff (nurses, midwives, and traditional birth attendants in contact with patient's blood). Young women also disproportionately engage in caregiving of infected children and adults and may thus be more exposed to infected fluids in this way compared to young men.

16. See Royce et al. 1997; Padian et al. 1997; Bolan et al. 1999 for developed country findings; and Mastro et al. 1994; Cameron et al. 1989; O'Farrell 2001; Gray et al. 2001 for developing country findings. See Boily et al. 2009 for meta-analysis of developed and developing country findings.

17. Fleming and Wasserheit 1999; Røttingen, Cameron, and Garnett 2001.

18. See Caldwell and Caldwell 1993; Weiss et al. 2000; Auvert et al. 2001.

19. The three prospective randomized controlled trials were conducted in Kisumu, Kenya (Bailey et al. 2007), Rakai, Uganda (Gray et al. 2007), and Orange Farm, South Africa (Auvert et al. 2005). Male circumcision has since been rolled out as a key HIV prevention strategy in several settings across sub-Saharan Africa.

20. See Boerma and Weir 2005.

21. KDHS 2010:86 among women aged 20–49 and men aged 20–54.

22. Gregson et al. 2002 for Zimbabwe and Pettifor et al. 2005 for South Africa.

23. It is worth noting that this might be part of the problem, as an article by Nnko et al. (2004) whose key argument is encapsulated by the title "Secretive Females or Swaggering Males" suggests. They argue and demonstrate that men typically exaggerate their reported number of sexual partners while women underreport. It is thus arguable whether young women's higher HIV rates might be signaling a greater number of partners regardless of what they report. However, this issue plagues all studies of sexual behavior based primarily on self-report (Hewett, Mensch, and Erulkar 2004; Fenton et al. 2001). Without access to biomarker data such as STI status, researchers often have to believe that people are telling the truth. Indeed, Nnko et al. (2004) were able to establish under-reporting by having HIV tests of the respondents available, and the investigators were able to see discrepancies between behavioral self-reports and HIV-prevalence levels.

24. For example, in Luo-Nyanza, 15–19-year-old male adolescents had an almost 3% HIV prevalence compared to an almost 29% HIV prevalence among 25–29-year-old men. (See figure 11 in chapter 4.) See Gouws et al. 2008 for similar age-gender prevalence patterns in several Southern African countries.

25. Glick and Sahn 2008; Bankole et al. 2009; Cleland, Ali and Shah 2006; Maharaj and Cleland 2005; Macphail and Campbell 2001; Lloyd 2005; Reynolds, Luseno, and Speizer 2012.

26. See Kretzschmar and Morris 1995; Morris et al. 1996; Halperin and Epstein 2004; Bearman, Moody, and Stovel 2004; Epstein 2007; Helleringer and Kohler 2007 for work on concurrent relationships, sexual networks, and HIV risk.

27. See, for example, Karanja 1994; Guyer 1994; Steady 1987; Booth 2003; Smith 2006; Hirsch et al. 2009.

28. Several surveys in different settings across the globe suggest widespread extramarital sex. In the United States, for example, between 20%–25% of men and 10%–15% of women report ever having extramarital sex (Laumann et al. 1994; Wiederman 1997). What varies is cultural acceptance of that behavior (Hirsch et al. 2009).

29. Reniers and Watkins 2010; Reniers and Tfaily 2012.

30. De Walque 2007; see also Eyawo et al. 2010.

31. Another critical feature above and beyond the individual decisions of young people is the stage of the HIV epidemic at which sexual networks in a community are operating. Once HIV is established in a population, the likelihood of an individual encountering HIV is much higher. For example if 10% of the population is HIV positive, an individual has a much higher likelihood of encountering an HIV-positive partner, compared to a population with a 0.5% prevalence, even if the number of sexual partners a person has had was the same. A preexisting STI epidemic might also serve as an accelerant for an HIV epidemic. In a study examining the HIV epidemic in four African cities, a key

contributing factor was an established herpes simplex virus (HSV-2) epidemic because there is an epidemiological synergy between prior STIs and the likelihood of getting HIV. Both kinds of epidemics are rapidly established when there is a high degree of concurrency in sexual networks. Buve et al. 2001; Glynn et al. 2001; Hitchcock and Fransen 1999; Fleming and Wasserheit 1999; Røttingen, Cameron, and Garnett 2001.

32. Lurie et al. 2003a, 2003b.

33. Carswell et al. 1989; Oruboloye, Caldwell, and Caldwell 1993; Mbugua et al. 1995. Nolen 2007; See also Nyanzi et al. 2004 for *boda boda* (bike taxi) men and HIV risk.

34. In a study in Thailand, Morris et al. (1996) found that bridge populations—people likely to have both high- and low-risk partners—can be critical in epidemics. Local women might have relationships with transient migrant workers such as truckers and a local man in their village or town, thus providing the sexual-network link between low- and high-risk populations.

35. Barnett and Whiteside 2002; Iliffe 2006; Mojola 2011a.

36. Barnett and Whiteside 2002; Vaughan 1991.

37. Nolen 2007.

38. UNDP 2013; KDHS 2010.

39. Ogot 2004.

40. In the KDHS for 2010, 63% and 62% of Nyanza's female and male inhabitants, respectively, were of Luo ethnicity. However, 84% and 85% of female and male HIV-positive cases, respectively, in Nyanza province were among people of Luo ethnicity.

41. In the last survey, the KDHS for 2004, in Kenya as a whole, 8.7% of women and 4.6% of men were HIV positive. However, in Nyanza province, 18.3% of women and 11.6% of men were HIV positive. These were the highest provincial rates in the country then. Among the Luo, 25.8% of women and 17.5% of men were HIV positive. While current statistics suggest slight reductions for women, rates for men are virtually unchanged. Response rates for HIV testing were 89% (91% for women, 87% for men). The continued high HIV rates suggest that the epidemic may have become endemic in this part of the country.

42. Barnett and Whiteside 2002; Pickering et al. 1997; Iliffe 2006; Pepin 2011.

43. Hunter, De Souza, and Twine 2008; Mojola 2011a.

44. At the time, there were 12 administrative districts in Nyanza province; however, four of them (Central Kisii, Gucha, Kuria, and Kisii North) were dominated by other ethnic groups (the Maasai, Kisii, and Luhya). Research in districts where those ethnic groups were dominant would have resulted in interviewing Luos who were likely to have assimilated to the lifestyles and traditions of other ethnic groups. Eight districts were predominantly Luo districts (Nyando, Bondo, Suba, Siaya, Rachuonyo, Migori, Kisumu, and Homa Bay [see also KDHS

2004])—what I call "Luo-Nyanza" in this book. (I first encountered this term in colloquial use in the field.) My fieldwork was in four of these districts.

45. See also Bondo, Kisumu, Nyando, and Homa Bay District Development Plans: Kenya n.d.

46. Kenya Education Directory 2006.

47. Key resources used in conducting interviews, writing field notes, and coding and analyzing data include Weiss (1994), van Maanen (1988), and Emerson, Fretz, and Shaw (1995), who draw on an inductive grounded theory approach to the process (Strauss and Corbin 1998; Charmaz 2001).

48. Luo names are often a combination of English or "Christian" names such as Mary, Jane, and George, and dhoLuo names such as Akinyi or Onyango. The pseudonyms I use in the book reflect this.

49. The KDHS for 2003 surveyed 8195 women (15–49) and 3578 men (15–54). HIV tests were conducted for 76% of the 4303 eligible women and 70% of the 4183 eligible men. Rural residents were more likely to be tested than urban residents (79% compared to 62%). In Nyanza province, however, 91.1% of women and 87% of men were tested. These represented the highest provincial response rates in the nation. The KDHS 2008–9 is a nationally representative household-based survey of 8444 women (15–49) and 3465 men (15–54). All the men and half the women were tested for HIV. HIV tests were conducted for 86% of the 4418 eligible women and 79% of the 3910 eligible men. Rural residents were more likely to be tested than urban residents (85% compared to 78%). In Nyanza province, however, 91% of women and 81% of men were tested. All analyses in this study are based on the sample of men and women tested for HIV.

## 2. CONSUMING WOMEN, MODERNITY, AND HIV RISK

1. See, for example, Vaughan (1991) on colonial discourses on African sexuality and their consequences for treatment of illness in East Africa, and the more recent debate about whether there is a coherent "African system of sexuality": see Caldwell, Caldwell, and Quiggin 1989; Ahlberg 1994; Heald 1995. Hill Collins (2004) discusses the exoticization of black sexuality in the United States. See Mbembé and Nuttall (2004) on the treatment of Africa as "other."

2. Ferguson 1999, 2006; Comaroff and Comaroff 2012:117.

3. Ankomah 1996, 1999; Cole 2004, 2010; Cornwall 2002; Dunkle et al. 2004; Hunter 2002, 2010; Kaufman and Stavrou 2004; Konde-Lule, Sewankambo, and Morris 1997; Leclerc-Madlala 2002, 2003; Longfield et al. 2004; Luke 2006, 2010; Meekers and Calvés 1997; Nyamnjoh 2005; Smith 2004; Swidler and Watkins 2007; Poulin 2007. See Luke and Kurz 2002; Luke 2003; Chatterji et al. 2004; and Leclerc-Madlala 2008 for reviews.

4. Nyamnjoh 2005 (West Africa); Cole 2005 (Madagascar); see also Cole 2010; Hunter 2002:112 (South Africa); see also Hunter 2010.

5. Transactional sex is also considered problematic because of its association with intimate partner violence, on the one hand, and HIV risk, on the other (Dunkle et al. 2004). Women's financial dependence on men makes them both more vulnerable within a relationship since they have little bargaining power and are more open to abuse. Intimate partner violence is not statistically linked to HIV risk in Kenya, however, unlike in other countries (Dude 2007). Indeed the 13% of young Luo women in Nyanza (15–29) who reported experiencing sexual violence in the KDHS for 2004 appeared to have almost four times lower rates of HIV (9.02%) than those who did not (34.54%). (For young women age 15–24, the difference is 0% to 40%.) Thus, the mechanisms for how the link between these three factors—transactional sex, intimate partner violence, and HIV risk—works is not apparent. This requires further, context-specific investigation. In Luo-Nyanza all three of these elements are strong features of the setting; however, they do not appear to be positively linked.

6. For example, in a study focused on 12 African countries using Demographic and Health Survey data, Parkhurst (2010) found that the richest women in Malawi, Tanzania, Kenya, Rwanda, Zambia, Cote d'Ivoire, Lesotho, and Uganda had the highest rates of HIV. (The wealth index is a five-item scale—1 = poorest, 2 = poor, 3 = middle, 4 = richer, 5 = richest—that is an asset-based measure of household wealth.) For Zimbabwe and Cameroon, it was middle-income and richer (but not the richest) women who had the highest rates. In Ghana, it was middle-income women who were most affected. Swaziland was the only exception, with the richest women having a 2% lower HIV prevalence rate compared to women of lower wealth quintiles. (Trends in Zimbabwe, Ghana, and Swaziland were not statistically significant, however.)

7. Fox 2010. See also Shelton, Cassell, and Adetunji 2005, and Mishra et al. 2007.

8. KDHS 2010:24–25.

9. My analysis of KDHS 2010.

10. Leclerc-Madlala 2003.

11. Hunter 2002:100–101.

12. Poulin 2007.

13. Luke and Kurz 2002:16; Moore, Biddlecom, and Zulu 2007.

14. Luke 2005.

15. Hunter 2002:101.

16. Ashforth 1999.

17. Mills and Ssewakiryanga 2005.

18. Ilouz 1997.

19. Zelizer 2000:818. The new term "commercial sex worker" moves toward a description of their labor, as opposed to a judgment of the morality of that labor.

It is striking that the clients, who are predominantly male, of sex workers, who are predominantly female, are not similarly morally judged when described as consumers of commercial sex. Wojcicki (2002) complicates even how commercial sex is viewed in her study of *ukuphanda*, informal sex work in urban South Africa.

20. Zelizer 2000:818; see also Zelizer 2005.

21. As Bernstein (2010) argues in her book, emotions are not necessarily absent in commercial sex, since the men in her study buying "the girlfriend experience" are also buying the emotional labor and companionship of a woman in addition to buying sex.

22. Chan 2006:47.

23. Epstein 1982.

24. O'Rourke 2007.

25. *Reuters*, August 30, 2011.

26. Mauss 1990; Zelizer 2005; Carruthers and Espeland 1998.

27. White 1990; Lurie et al. 2003a, 2003b; Nolen 2007; Pepin 2011.

28. White 1990; Ferguson 1999.

29. Yngstrom 2002; Daley and Englert 2010; Arbache, Kolev, and Filipiak 2010; Chu 2011; Dworkin et al. 2012; Mojola 2014.

30. Coontz 2005; Eisenstein 2009.

31. Budig and England 2001; Hodges and Budig 2010.

32. Shipton 2007.

33. Rubin 1975.

34. Sometimes, however, the wealth was raised by a slightly older, working young man, or from the proceeds from his sister's marriage.

35. Silberschmidt 1992, 2001, 2004; Hunter 2002, 2010; Ashforth 1999; Mojola 2014.

36. Swidler and Watkins 2007:157.

37. See Parry and Bloch 1989 for the role of money exchange in upholding social-structural reproduction.

38. Weiss 1993.

39. McGowan 2006; Burke 1996; Griffin 2004.

40. Friedman 2001:159.

41. Burke 1996:136 ("for," "within": emphasis in the original; "new needs": my emphasis).

42. Coontz 2005; Cherlin 2009.

43. Zukin and Maguire 2004:175.

44. Bailey 1989:75.

45. See also Veblen 2006.

46. Thomas 2008:115.

47. Weinbaum et al. 2008:18.

48. Thomas 2008:100.

49. Thomas 2008:105.

50. Bailey 1989.

51. Cherlin 2009; Bailey 1989.

52. Cherlin 2009:71.

53. Bailey 1989:72.

54. McRobbie 1997:74.

55. Woodruffe 1997.

56. Harris 2004:165.

57. Harris 2004:166.

58. Sobek 1997; U.S. Census Bureau 2012.

59. Bureau of Labor Statistics 2013.

60. Veblen (2006) argued that wives' consumption practices were in fact "duties," a way of "putting in evidence [a husband's] ability to sustain large pecuniary damage without impairing his superior opulence" (40). Indeed, the wife as the "ceremonial consumer of goods which he produces" (57) was demonstrating to the world the respectability and repute of the family as being able to engage in conspicuous consumption as part of the leisure class.

61. Nyamnjoh 2005:317.

## 3. HISTORICAL AND CULTURAL CONTEXT

Epigraph: Eckholm 1977:18–19.

1. These rates were no doubt exacerbated by the AIDS epidemic. Table A1 in the appendix shows infant mortality rates in Nyanza over the last three decades compared to Kenya as a whole.

2. Cohen and Atieno Odhiambo 1989.

3. Barnett and Whiteside 2002; Pickering et al. 1997; Iliffe 2006.

4. Negin et al. 2010; Gargano et al. 2012. Gargano et al. also found that between 2003 and 2008, 55.5% of adult deaths in one HDSS in Nyanza covering 140,000 residents were attributable to HIV/AIDS. See also Yamano and Jayne 2005.

5. According to Bicego, Rutstein, and Johnson (2003), in 1998, Kenya had 1.2 million orphans. Of these, 9.3% of under-15 youth were single orphans (who had lost one parent) and 0.9% were double orphans (who had lost both parents). By 2004, Kenya had 1.5 million orphans of whom 388,064 lived in Nyanza province. This means that Nyanza has 25% of Kenya's orphans. See Mishra and Bignami-Van Assche 2008.

6. Many child-headed homes have sprung up in the wake of the epidemic. These are homes with no adults present. They typically occur when one parent and then another dies. The latter is often cared for by the oldest child, who is then left to take care of the remaining children. The length of the epidemic has meant that homes that would earlier have accommodated orphans can no longer

do so; they are full. This results in no place for children to go when their parents die. Typically, adults in the community, community health workers, government social workers, or nongovernmental organizations step in to help with resources, food, and school fees. See, for example, Bicego et al. 2003; Nolen 2007.

7. Evans-Pritchard 1935.

8. Ocholla Ayayo 1997; Muriungi 2005:177. See Geissler and Prince 2010 for a more extensive discussion of *chira*.

9. Potash 1986; Cohen and Atieno Odhiambo 1989; Nyambedha et al. 2003; Shipton 2007; Geissler and Prince 2010; Agot et al. 2010; Mojola 2014.

10. Okeyo and Allen 1994; Shipton 2007; Ayikukwei et al. 2008; Mojola 2014.

11. See also Shipton 2007 and Geissler and Prince 2010 for discussion of various sex-related customs.

12. Ogot 2004.

13. See Shipton 2007 for descriptions and discussion of Luo funerals, especially how they were traditionally run before large-scale AIDS mortality. See also Geissler and Prince 2010.

14. Mojola 2014.

15. See also Njue, Voeten, and Remes 2009.

16. For excellent and detailed ethnographies and books on the Luo, see Whisson 1964; DuPré 1968; Parkin 1978; Shipton 1989; Cohen and Atieno Odhiambo 1989; Shipton 2007; Ogot 2009; and Geissler and Prince 2010. I draw on these sources, as well as my own fieldwork and interviews among middle-aged and older adults, in this chapter.

17. See also Dupré 1968; Shipton 2007.

18. Whisson 1964; Ominde 1987; Cohen and Atieno Odhiambo 1989.

19. Whisson 1964; Ominde 1987; Cohen and Atieno Odhiambo 1989. Unlike many other ethnic groups in Kenya, the Luo did not have initiation ceremonies where youth were sequestered and taught the customs, beliefs, and practices of their community before being released through a variety of rituals that marked them as recognized adults. Neither boys nor girls were circumcised. In some areas within Luoland, however, a ritual that was sometimes performed that marked adulthood was the removal of six front teeth. Respondents noted that this was primarily for medicinal reasons; when a person got sick, gaps in the teeth allowed the insertion of medicine into the mouth of a patient whose mouth might otherwise be tightly closed. However, while this surgery was performed, the participant's ability to remain quiet during the ordeal was considered a sign of maturity and adulthood. Thus, some among the older generations of Luo have gaps in their teeth (*singare*). See also Ochieng 1979; Bailey et al. 2002.

20. Whisson 1964; Blount 1973; Malo 1999; see also Cohen and Atieno Odhiambo 1989.

21. As a man could not marry a woman from his own clan (essentially any of the girls he grew up with who were in his compound or his neighborhood), many

of these socializing opportunities were to enable youth from different clan groups to meet.

22. Evans-Pritchard 1950; Malo 1999; Whisson 1964; Shipton 2007.

23. Whisson 1964:57.

24. While this story was recounted several times, I did not meet any women to whom this actually happened.

25. Now, however, the older women told me, giving birth before marriage is seen as a sign of fertility. The logic behind this would be that in an age where polygamy is increasingly expensive, and parenthood remains an important marker of adulthood for men, barrenness has become more problematic. Thus, a woman who has proven fertile once provides proof that she can bear her future husband's children. This is why they believed young men were now said to marry single mothers without the sanctions of the past.

26. See Stewart 2001 and Kaler 2001 for accounts of similar discrepancies between elder reports of the past and the reality in Uganda and Malawi.

27. Statistics use data from KDHS 2004 for women aged 30–49 and for men 30–59.

28. Blount 1973; Whisson 1964:50, 53. The Luo are organized into clans segmented by genealogical lineage. They are patrilineal and virilocal. See also Hay 1976.

29. In some cases, however, this was not a mock struggle, and the force was genuine. This is both recorded in Hay (1976:94–95) as well as in a few accounts in my interviews among older women who said they were forced into marriage.

30. Mboya and Achieng 2001; Cohen and Atieno Odhiambo 1989; Shipton 2007.

31. Evans-Pritchard 1950:234–35.

32. Shipton 1989; Ferguson 1992, 1994.

33. Comaroff and Comaroff 2006:113.

34. Evans-Pritchard 1950.

35. Ocholla-Ayayo 1977:40.

36. Evans-Pritchard 1950:206.

37. Arnold 1981.

38. DuPré 1968; Whisson 1964; Cohen and Atieno Odhiambo 1989; Hay 1976. This might be accompanied by a familiar population-ecological story: as population density and thus agricultural intensity across family plots of land increased on the hills, the quality of soil declined. Further, erosion of topsoil over time due to a lack of proper drainage in many areas also affected the productivity of the soil. Thus, the shift toward the lake might also have been a shift to finding more space to live as well as more agriculturally productive land.

39. Shipton 1989; Fearn 1961.

40. Whisson 1964:i; see also Odinga 1967; DuPré 1968:22; Shipton 1989, 2007.

41. DuPré 1968; Hay 1976; Shipton 1989; Cohen and Atieno Odhiambo 1989.

42. Cohen and Atieno Odhiambo 1989.

43. Hay 1976.

44. Cohen and Atieno Odhiambo 1989:112.

45. Cohen and Atieno Odhiambo 1989:113.

46. Cohen and Atieno Odhiambo 1989:113; see also Fearn 1961:90, 111–13, 147.

47. Malo 1999:31.

48. Malo 1999:31.

49. Cohen and Atieno Odhiambo 1989:114.

50. Merton 1968.

51. Atieno Odhiambo 2001.

52. Mboya 2012:275.

53. Odinga 1967:76–77.

54. Mboya 2012.

55. Interestingly, this perspective distinctively echoes Thorstein Veblen, writing in 1899, on the growth of conspicuous consumption in the transition to leisure societies. He argued that, in the leisure class, "unproductive consumption of goods is honorable, primarily as a mark of prowess and a perquisite of human dignity" (2006:43).

56. Cohen and Atieno Odhiambo 1989:122.

57. See also Bogonko 1992, for similar perspectives in Kenya as a whole.

58. Kenyan school at the time consisted of seven years of primary (elementary) school (Standard 1 to Standard 7) and six years of secondary (high) school (Form 1 to Form 6). Currently, it consists of eight years of primary school (Standard 1 to Standard 8) and four years of secondary school (Form 1 to Form 4).

59. In the KDHS for 2004, for respondents over 30 years of age, among Luo respondents in Nyanza only 14.5% of women had no education, while in the rest of the country 23% had no education. However, 45% dropped out in primary school. As a result, while only 16% of Luo women entered secondary school, 23% of non-Luo/Nyanza women entered.

60. This decision might sometimes be tied to family needs—for example, a brother ready to marry needing the cows contracted through his sister's marriage. See also Shipton 2007 for how young women were seen as entrustments available to a family as a strategy to gain access to wealth, especially in times of dire poverty.

61. I was not able to verify whether young women still lived with Pim. While Pim was discussed frequently in interviews with older women, Pim was not mentioned once in interviews with young women. Young women's living arrangements when discussed were typically with parents or other relatives. Some orphan girls stayed with their grandmother, but they did not refer to her as Pim. This suggests that this is a tradition that is dying or has died out.

62. Bogonko 1992; Setel 1995; Day 1998; Stambach 2000; Mbugua 2007; Shipton 2007.

63. Statistics calculated from KDHS 2004 among male respondents over 30, comparing non-Luo men to Luo men residing in Nyanza province.

64. Bogonko 1992; Lelei and Weidman 2012; Hornsby 2012.

65. Odinga 1967:7.

66. See also Baker and Jimerson 1992.

67. Shipton 2007.

68. Shipton 1989:24.

69. Shipton 1989:51–52.

70. Geissler and Prince 2010.

71. See Swidler 1986, 2001 for discussion of cultural toolkit and cultural reportoires.

72. See Maurer 2006 for a review.

73. Simmel 2004.

74. Bloch and Parry 1989, Keister 2002.

75. Bloch and Parry 1989:1–2.

76. Bloch and Parry 1989:14.

77. Bingenheimer 2007; Ferguson 1992.

78. Bloch and Parry 1989:2.

79. Shipton 1989.


4. LOVE, MONEY, AND HIV PREVENTION

Epigraph: Clark 2004:158.

1. Mojola and Everett 2012.

2. Bogle 2008; England, Fitzgibbons Shafer, and Fogarty 2007; Wolfe 2000; Glenn and Marquandt 2001.

3. Table A2 in the appendix illustrates the HIV prevalence among young Luo-Nyanza women and men, by age group with 95% confidence intervals and sample sizes. As the table illustrates, differences among teenagers do not have overlapping confidence intervals, but rates at other ages do. That is, teenage girls' rates are significantly different from the rates of teenage boys, but not significantly different from those of men at older ages. This highlights their reduced risk of getting HIV from same-aged partners compared to getting it from men who are older.

4. Assuming minimal importance of biological factors, or a counterbalancing of young women's physiological vulnerability with Luo men's lack of circumcision.

5. Clark, Kabiru, and Mathur 2010.

6. Glynn et al. 2001; Zabin and Kiragu 1998; Clark 2004. See also Hirsch et al. 2002, 2009.

7. It is worth noting that the median age at sexual debut has not changed: every age group from 15–19 to 45–49 had a median age of sexual debut of 15, and only one-third of 15- to 19-year-olds were virgins. This illustrates that this has been characteristic among Luo women for the last few decades. Median age at marriage for women above age 30 has not changed either, with the exception of those aged 40–44 who had a median age of 16. Women aged 25–29 had a median age at marriage of 18, suggesting that the median age at marriage may be rising. These statistics are important because they tell us that while the perceptions and consequences of early sex and marriage are changing, the timing of the practices themselves has not changed much. The median age at first sex for Luo-Nyanza men was age 15, which was similar to women; however, the median age at first marriage was 22, five years older than women. By age 32, 95% of men were married. Thus, many men had a longer premarital period compared to women.

8. Clark 2004; of course, marriage was also clearly a risk factor for men. However, no teenage boys reported marriage.

9. Boily et al. 2009.

10. See also Poulin 2007.

11. Terms such as "eating," "food," or "consumption" are common metaphors used in this and many African settings. For example, *The Politics of the Belly,* the title of a famous book by Jean-Francois Bayart, referring to how corruption works; people's reference to getting a piece of the "national cake," referring to wanting a portion of state resources; discussions about how corrupt politicians have "eaten"; and so on. Here, Macy's reference to "eating" the man means the girl's taking up with him so that she can "eat" or consume his money.

12. Hunter 2002, 2010; Poulin 2007; Swidler and Watkins 2007.

13. See also Agnew 1994 and Cole 2004, 2010.

14. Fine 1988. Michelle Fine discusses the silencing of discourse of female desire within institutional settings such as schools in the United States. When female sexuality was discussed, it was in the context of negative outcomes such as sexual violence against women, as opposed to positive outcomes such as sexual pleasure.

15. Clark, Kabiru, and Mathur 2010.

16. For other settings, see, for example, Flood 2003; Watkins 2004; MacPhail and Campbell 2001; Poulin 2007; Ankomah 1999; Tavory and Swidler 2009. It is puzzling and perhaps should be studied in its own right how a uniform attitude, expressed with uniform phrases, across many countries, can be formed toward a product (that is, such negative attitudes are not broadcast to the same degree as advertisements in support of the product), unless, of course, they are uniformly true.

17. Among unmarried men, 65% of 15- to 19-year-olds and 81% of 20- to 24-year-olds reported condom use; see also Watkins 2004.

18. See Luke 2003:321–22 for critique of these assumptions.

19. Flood 2003; Smith 2004.

20. Halperin and Epstein 2004.

21. Clark, Kabiru, and Mathur 2010.

22. Luke et al. 2011. In an earlier survey of the same site, Nancy Luke (2005) found a significant negative relationship between condom use and the level of transfer (regardless of whether it was money or gifts). That is, the more women received from their partner, the less likely they were to use condoms. The study concluded that "adolescent girls and older women are active agents who make conscious trade-offs between the risks and benefits of informal exchange relationships" (2005:345). Indeed, safe sex may not necessarily be a positive or desired option for a young woman in a relationship with a man who is demonstrating that he can provide now—and therefore potentially later—and in a context where demonstrated fertility might provide the impetus for the man in question to marry her.

23. Flood 2003:363. See also Tavory and Swidler 2009.

24. See also Ankomah 1999; Mills and Ssewakiryanga 2005.

25. See also Luke et al. 2011.

26. For similar contradictions, see also Haram 1995 for Tanzania, and Bledsoe 1990 for Sierra Leone.

27. Mojola 2011b.

28. See Harrison 2008 for relationship hiding among young South African women.

29. Using DHS data from several African countries, Fox 2010 illustrates the higher HIV rates of wealthier men. In my own analysis of the KDHS 2010, this is also the case, not just among all men, but also among men under 30 years.

30. Luke 2005.

31. Young women did sometimes marry men considerably older than themselves; however, this was not their ideal when they talked about it.

32. Part of this was also that older girls (for example, out of school or in their late teens and early 20s) were more realistic about their marriage prospects and were willing to settle for a man who was working, even if he did not make very much money. By that time, they were also more likely to have started some income-generating activity of their own and thus were less dependent on a man than when they were teenagers.

33. See also Smith 2006; Hirsch et al. 2009.

34. Hamilton and Armstrong (2009) found that hooking up serves a similar function for young college women in the United States, allowing them to have a sexual relationship without the emotional attachment that might distract them from school.

35. Mojola 2011b.

36. See also Ashforth 1999; Hunter 2010.

37. An interesting circularity then arose where consuming women could attract wealthy men, who in turn could afford to maintain consuming women.

38. See also Watkins 2004.

39. Someone classed as a "serious Christian" was someone who had abandoned their cultural beliefs and practices. See also Geissler and Prince 2010.

40. See also Swidler and Watkins 2007; Brenner 1998.

41. In Malawi, Watkins 2004; Schatz 2005; Smith and Watkins 2005; and Reniers 2008 illustrate how before antiretroviral drugs were largely available, and when HIV status was unknown, local Malawians used a combination of strategies to manage their exposure to HIV risk such as discussion with suspected unfaithful spouses, the use of social networks to find out information about potential spouses or the behavior of a current spouse, confronting extramarital partners directly, and separating from or divorcing the unfaithful spouse among both women and men.

42. Kabiru et al. (2010), studying youth aged 18–26 in Kisumu, found that 64% of women and 55% of men had had at least one HIV test in the last ten years.

43. In the survey, HIV test results were not released to respondents. Instead, respondents were directed to nearby facilities for voluntary counseling and testing (VCT). These were the primary means for people to find out their HIV status. The big assumption here, of course, is that the results of the previous test on which they reported and the survey test matched.

44. Table A3 in the appendix illustrates the 2004 KDHS HIV-prevalence rates among young Luo-Nyanza women and men by age group. Of note is the tripling in rates among teenage girls and boys between the surveys in 2004 and 2010. (See table A2 in the appendix for 2010 rates.) It is also worth noting that young women's rates between ages 15 and 24 were significantly different from those of same-aged men (that is, there were no overlapping intervals).

45. For women who have never had children, 38% of 15- to 19-year-olds and 52% of 20- to 24-year-olds have ever been tested; for women who have had at least one child, 89% of 15- to 19-year-olds and 89% of 20- to 24-year-olds have ever been tested.

46. Kabiru et al. 2010.

47. See Yeatman 2007 for a review of studies examining the links between HIV testing, self-reported sexual behavior change, and STI/HIV incidence.

48. Eyawo et al. 2010.

## 5. SCHOOL AND THE PRODUCTION OF CONSUMING WOMEN

1. Gregson et al. 2001; Fox 2012.

2. Glynn et al. 2004.

3. Fortson 2008.

4. Gregson et al. 2001; de Walque et al. 2005; Hargreaves et al. 2008; Jukes, Simmons, and Bundy 2008.

5. De Walque et al. 2005; Pettifor et al. 2008. Preliminary analysis of the KDHS data for 2004 and 2010 suggests that these dynamics may be starting to play out in Kenya. In the KDHS for 2004, for example, among all women, those with no formal education had the lowest rates of HIV, with a nonlinear increase in HIV rates at different levels of education. Young women under 30 with the highest level of education had the highest rates of HIV. In the KDHS for 2010, while, among all women, those with no formal education still had the lowest rates of HIV, among young women those with primary education had the highest rates, and those with at least some postprimary education had slightly lower rates of HIV. However, and critically, none of these trends is statistically significant, or at least not yet. Among Luo-Nyanza young women, the trends are particularly puzzling. As noted earlier, every young woman surveyed had some formal education. Women with the highest education had the highest rates of HIV, followed by women with incomplete primary education. Women with complete primary and incomplete secondary school had the next highest rates. Those who completed secondary school, however, had the lowest rates. See Pettifor et al. 2008 for comparison with this last result.

6. Ross and Wu 1995; Caldwell 1980; Jejheeboy 1995; Bledsoe et al. 1998; Lloyd et al. 2000; Johnson-Hanks 2006.

7. Stambach 2000; Vavrus 2003.

8. See also Jukes, Simmons, and Bundy 2008.

9. See note 5.

10. Lloyd et al. 2000.

11. Buchmann 1999; Bradshaw 1993; Hughes 1994.

12. Fuller 1991:4; Hughes 1994.

13. Fuller 1991:xvii.

14. Bogonko 1992; Buchmann 1999; Mwiria 1991; Whitehead 1993; Branch 2011; Lelei and Weidman 2012.

15. Somerset 2011.

16. KDHS 1989.

17. The total fertility rates (TFR) that produced the current family sizes of the youth in this book were 7.1 children per woman between 1983 and 1985, and 6.9 children per woman between 1986 and 1988 (KDHS 1989:22). Current fertility rates in Nyanza are 5.4 children per woman (KDHS 2010).

18. Ngau 1987; Mwiria 1990; Nzomo 1989; Hornsby 2012.

19. Bradshaw 1993; see also Bogonko 1992.

20. Muya 2000.

21. Somerset 2011.

22. Hornsby 2012.

23. Bradshaw 1993; Buchmann 1999; Beoku-Betts 1998; Lelei 2005; Eloundou-Enyegue and Davanzo 2003; Somerset 2011; Colclough and Webb 2012.

24. Lelei 2005; Ngware et al. 2006; Kakubo-Mariara and Mwabu 2007.

25. Bold et al. 2013; Nishimura and Yamano 2012.

26. Statistics from an analysis of the level of educational attainment among the 15–24-year-old Luo of Nyanza province compared to other Kenyans using data from the Kenya Demographic and Health Survey (KDHS 2010).

27. Since this is cross-sectional data, these percentages reflect the highest educational attainment of the respondents at the time of interview. This means that particularly among women under 30 years of age, they do not reflect intentions, for example, to return to school if their educational attainment was stated as incomplete. Since many of these decisions to drop out or return to school are made processually (Johnson-Hanks 2006), whether a woman will return to school is uncertain at a given point in time, even if she is currently at home (that is, in the sample of those over 30, a "dropping out" designation is more straightforward).

28. Examining youth aged 15–29 does not show much change in these trends, that is, even accounting for delayed age for grade (Mensch and Lloyd 2001). Comparable statistics for this sample include that 64% men and 73% women of Luo-Nyanza 15- to 29-year-olds had no more than primary education compared to 55% and 63% of men and women, respectively, in Kenya as a whole. For high school, similar percentages of Luo-Nyanza 15- to 29-year-olds had completed high school, compared to 14% and 19% of women and men in Kenya.

29. Even accounting for the additional years it takes to get in to higher education by looking at accomplishments by age 29, these numbers had barely budged among Luo-Nyanza youth: 2.7% of women and 4.8% of men reported higher education. Among non-Luo-Nyanza youth, there was a 1%–2% increase. 6.9% of women and 7.8% of men reported higher education.

30. See also Lelei and Wiedman 2012.

31. Cohen and Atieno Odhiambo 1989.

32. Hornsby 2012; Branch 2011.

33. UNDP 2005.

34. Lelei and Weidman 2012; Bold et al. 2013; Nishimura and Yamano 2012.

35. During the period of study, the exchange rate ranged from US $1 to 70–72 Kenyan shillings. The value of US currency is based on the rate of US $1 to 70 Kenya shillings.

36. In light of this, it is worth noting that the secondary-school youth interviewed for this study represent the select few who not only had managed to be smart enough to get a secondary-school place, but also were fortunate enough to have parents, relatives, guardians, or donors able to support them through school. (That is, the fact that they were present in school on the day of interviewing meant that they were likely to have paid their fees; otherwise they would have been sent home.)

37. By some estimates, the majority of the education budget (75%) goes to teacher salaries.

38. Mojola 2011b.

39. Bennell 2005; Nyambedha, Wandibba, and Aagaard-Hansen 2003; and Kakooza and Kimuna 2005.

40. Muyanga et al. (2010) found a decrease in grade progression in the mid-2000s. This was associated with the lower educational attainment and income of the household head. They further found that the transition from primary to secondary school was positively associated with living with parents (as opposed to other relatives), household head income and educational attainment, and lower household dependency ratios.

41. Corporal punishment in Kenyan schools was a regular practice until a recent ban.

42. Evans, Kremer, and Ngatia 2009; Duflo et al. 2006.

43. Buchmann 1999; Dore 1976.

44. Tracer studies track a cohort of students in the years following graduation to examine the rate of job uptake. See Buchmann 1999; Dore 1976.

45. Ngware et al. 2006, Agesa and Agesa 2002; Mojola 2011b.

46. See also Mojola 2014.

47. Paterson 2006:27.

48. Brown 1990.

49. Pugh 2009.

50. Fearn 1961.

51. See Sommer 2009, 2010, for discussions on Tanzanian schoolgirl challenges in managing menstruation while pursuing school, including the expense of sanitary pads, limited education from their parents about menstruation, and logistical challenges such as limited water in schools.

52. Brint 2006.

53. Serpell 1993; Carter 1999; Stambach 2000.

54. Fuller 1991:96.

55. Fuller 1991; Serpell 1993; Stambach 2000; Carter 1999.

56. Swidler 1986, 2001.

57. See also Mojola 2011b.

58. Mojola 2011b.

59. Bledsoe (1990) illustrates this process among those in Sierra Leone who pay school fees for schoolgirls with parents' approval, in the hope of marrying them later.

60. See, for example, Bledsoe 1990; Komba-Malekela and Liljeström 1994; Kelly 2000; Mensch and Lloyd 2001; Leach et al. 2003; Nyamnjoh 2005.

61. See Swidler and Watkins (2007) for a description of these "ties of dependence." This point is not trivial since a lack of goodwill between the school and the community could lead to running battles between the two. In one school, for example, conflict between the principal and the community led to the sabotaging of school facilities by community members. An attempt to set up a system to

pipe water into the school would mean that the school would no longer hire locals to carry water to the school, and these locals would thus lose money. So the pipe was sabotaged on several occasions.

62. While I was unable to verify this particular story (the student did not want to name the school specifically), it is plausible according to both the HIV rates in population-based surveys in the area and the many accounts related to me of teacher-student relationships.

63. During fieldwork, I encountered many urban legends that once people found out about their positive HIV status, regardless of gender or occupation, they would attempt to sleep with as many people as possible because they "don't want to die alone." Stories would often feature an individual who on dying would leave behind a list of all the potential victims. Thus, this statement was a "teacher version" of this larger perception of people living with HIV. According to the KDHS from 2010, however, HIV-positive people are more likely to use condoms compared to HIV-negative people.

64. In the KDHS from 2004, 8.1% of male Kenyan teachers were HIV positive compared to 4.6% of male nonteachers; in Luo-Nyanza, male teachers also had twice the rate of nonteachers, though the sample sizes were very small. See also Bennell 2003.

65. Kiragu et al. 2006.

66. Jessor 1991:602.

67. Jessor 1991:603.

68. See Frye 2012 for a discussion of a version of this sequential model at work among schoolgirls in Malawi.

69. I will admit that this was a role I embraced. Once interviews were over, I switched off the tape recorder and invited students to quiz me, in an effort to, in an albeit small way, reverse the power dynamics inherent in interviews. Many questions were about how I had ended up a graduate student in America. Many of my responses followed this sequential model: telling them my life story, emphasizing how hard I worked and how much I had sacrificed to get to that point, including setting aside relationships with boys, and how much family support I had had along the way. In one of the schools, the principal asked me to speak at their speech day. In that speech, I talked about young women's high HIV risk, encouraged girls to work hard, and told them that they were just as smart as their male counterparts (as many had received the message that they were not as smart as boys), and I encouraged parents to continue to support their daughters' education and reminded them of the value of that education.

70. In the United States, the combination model seems normative, but is supported by more widespread access to condoms and birth control, greater parental ability to financially support school-going children, and greater availability of part-time jobs for high school students.

71. This and the next case study were not tape-recorded; instead, I took detailed notes during the interviews and wrote them up afterward. I have placed quotation marks around verbatim quotes and summarized the rest of their interview in these descriptions.

72. See Mojola 2014 for young men out of school who pursued nonnormative transactional relationships with widows and rich older women.

73. Mojola 2011b.

74. In a paper, I draw on McNeely and Barber's (2010) definition of how parents make adolescents feel loved. They highlight three dimensions of supportive parenting: emotional support, instrumental support, and informational support. I argue there that orphan girls who felt loved based on these dimensions were less likely to engage in transactional relationships with older men than those who lacked either financial provision or emotional support. See Mojola 2011b.

75. Bearman et al. 2004.

## 6. GENDERED ECONOMIES AND THE ROLE OF ECOLOGY IN HIV RISK

1. Charles 1992; Williams 1992; Reskin 1993; Charles and Bradley 2009.

2. Campbell 1997; Hunter 2002, 2010; Mojola 2011a.

3. Mojola 2011a.

4. Chant and Jones 2005; Canagarajah and Nielsen 2001.

5. Eisemon and Schwille 1991:26.

6. See also Stambach 2000; Vavrus 2003.

7. Osler 1993.

8. Frye 2012. See also Kabiru et al. 2013 on how African youth cope with the disjuncture between aspirations and reality.

9. I provide data up to the age of 29 in order to capture most youth who were out of school (that is, most were likely to have finished school by age 29). An important caveat here is that the survey does not allow us to parse out who is still in school and who is not. However, many youth in interviews noted that it was impossible for them to be both in school and at work. The two were seen as incompatible. From the on-the-ground point of view, youth currently working were likely out of school. Women were more likely to work if they were married or had ever been married (for example, widowed or divorced) than if they had never been married. For figure 12, the following are the *totals* for each group among youth age 15–29. Age-specific group rates and sample sizes in parentheses are: Kenyan women 43% (2227); Kenyan men 77.9% (1677); Luo-Nyanza women 47.2% (254); Luo-Nyanza men 66.1% (199).

10. Omolo (2012), drawing on 2005–6 data from the Kenyan Labor Force Survey, comes to the same conclusion about gender differences in the relative

participation of women and men when focusing on labor-force participation rates (the ratio of the labor force to the overall size of the cohort), a different measure of employment, among Kenyan youth, especially among those in their 20s. Specifically, he finds that 30% of both male and female 15- to 19-year-olds, 73% and 68% of male and female 20- to 24-year-olds, and 93% and 82% of male and female 25- to 29-year-olds participate in the labor force. Labor-force inactivity is defined as voluntary (being at home or in school) and involuntary (unable to find work).

11. The extent to which education changes or improves prospects for young people in other parts of Africa is worth exploring in a little detail. Al-Samarrai and Bennell (2007) showed that, rather than being a blanket disadvantage for all youth, the employment reality varied by level of education. In their analysis of the job markets in four African countries (Malawi, Uganda, Tanzania, and Zimbabwe), they noted inadequate growth in the formal sector and a decline in wage employment as a proportion of the labor force, which seems to support the widespread belief that those educated past primary school are unable to find appropriate employment. However, they reported the results of nearly complete cohort tracer studies conducted in the four countries, tracing those who leave secondary school and university graduates from up to 20 years earlier. In 2001, 83%–94% of university graduates were in wage employment. However, for those who leave junior and senior secondary school, only 39% and 54%, respectively, were in wage employment in Tanzania and Uganda, while 23%–35% were undertaking further full-time education and training. Of those searching for wage employment in Tanzania, after 6.5 years, only 35%–40% had found jobs. As a result, there were increased levels of self-employment among those who left secondary school. The challenge is that these data are based on all cohorts across all years, and were thus not broken into cohort specific employment rates; that is, the job market could have been good for older generations of those who left secondary school but worse for younger generations, but we do not know this from the data.

12. See note 29 in chapter 5.

13. See also Setel 1999.

14. They could have used report forms from schools to prove the number of years of schooling, but these were not the same as national certificates.

15. Geheb and Binns 1997; Bryceson 2002.

16. As noted in chapter 3, many households were caring for multiple orphans. Many made ends meet through a combination of subsistence farming for food, hand-me-downs for clothes, borrowing from extended family relatives, and engaging in multiple livelihoods with household members pooling income from different small businesses.

17. Table A4 in the appendix shows both results specific to age groups and results for all young women under 30. As the table illustrates, working young women aged 15–29 have significantly higher HIV-prevalence rates compared to nonworking young women (that is, there are no overlapping confidence

intervals). However, the trends specific to age groups are not significant. While they trend in the same direction, they have overlapping confidence intervals.

18. I discuss these programs in more detail in chapter 7.

19. These are groups where every member contributes monthly money to a communal fund, and every month a member gets the sum total to do their project.

20. Okoko 2000; Mail and Guardian 2007.

21. Kearns 1993; MacIntyre and Ellaway 2000.

22. Acheson 1981; Thompson 1985; Steady 1987; Stirrat 1989; Carsten 1989; Geheb and Binns 1997; Seeley and Allison 2005; Merten and Haller 2007; Béné and Merten 2008; Mojola 2011a.

23. Mojola 2011a.

24. Mojola 2011a.

25. Mojola 2011b.

26. See also Mojola 2011b.

27. Mojola 2011a.

28. Geheb and Binns 1997; Njiru et al. 2006; Odada, Ochola, and Olago 2009; Okoko 2000; Ong'or and Long-Cang 2007; Sikoyo and Goldman 2007; Njiru et al. 2008; MDG Center 2009.

29. Njiru et al. 2008; Sikoyo and Goldman 2007; Kateregga and Sterner 2009.

30. Mojola 2011a.

31. These sorts of relationships between fishermen and fisherwomen have been documented in other settings throughout the continent. See Béné and Merten 2008 for a review.

32. There were thriving commercial sex businesses in several fishing towns, and there were several women who exclusively sold sex to fishermen, and some who combined commercial sex work with work in the fishing industry. These were distinct from *jaboya* relationships.

33. Mojola 2011a.

34. Mojola 2011a; Kwena et al. 2012; Camlin, Kwena, and Dworkin 2013.

35. Lurie et al. 2003a, 2003b; Campbell 2003; Hunter 2002, 2010; Nolen 2007.

## 7. "TO STEM HIV IN AFRICA, PREVENT TRANSMISSION TO YOUNG WOMEN"

1. See also Gouws et al. 2008; Clark 2004.

2. While male circumcision does not reduce transmission of HIV to women, a lower HIV-prevalence pool of partners for young women will mean they are less likely to encounter HIV-positive partners.

3. Stewart, Powell, and Greer 2009. See http://news.yahoo.com/startups-cup-helps-kenyan-girls-stay-school-172721776.html.

4. Baird et al. 2010, 2011, 2012.

5. Mojola 2011a.

6. Kim et al. 2008; Dworkin and Blankenship 2009.

7. Erulkar et al. 2006.

8. Epstein 2007; Dunbar et al. 2010.

9. Pronyk et al. 2006; Pronyk et al. 2008.

10. Pyle and Ward 2003; Eisenstein 2009; see also Ferguson 2006 for spread of nongovernmental organizations.

11. See www.oecd.org/development/povertyreduction/48869464.pdf.

12. Mojola 2011a.

13. Hansen 1999; Leclerc-Madlala 2003; Nyamnjoh 2005; Cole 2010.


EPILOGUE

1. UNAIDS 2012.

2. As of December 2011, according to WHO/UNAIDS/UNICEF; see www.who.int/hiv/data/ART_coverage_2011.png.

3. See Padian et al. 2011 for review of biomedical developments.

4. Quinn et al. 2000; Royce et al. 1997.

5. Eyawo et al. 2010; Chemaitelly and Abu-Raddad 2013; Hugonnet et al. 2002.

6. De Walque 2005; Eyawo et al. 2010.

7. Cohen et al. 2011.

8. Baeten et al. 2012. The study found a 67% relative risk reduction among those given Viread (TDF) and a 75% among those given Truvada (TDF-FTC), a combination ARV drug. Robert Grant and colleagues (2010) gave FTC-TDF to sero-negative men who have sex with men and found they had a 44% reduction in HIV incidence compared to men taking a placebo. Among men with high adherence, in whom there were detectable levels of the drug, there was a 92% relative HIV risk reduction.

9. A qualitative study nested within the Baeten et al. (2012) study by Ware et al. (2012) reported that after experiencing a "discordance dilemma"—where participants found an incompatibility between staying healthy and staying together, and between loving and wanting to have sex with their partner and being hurt by their infidelity and wanting to preserve their life—the participants found that the drug was a way to keep the relationship going. Adherence to the drug then became an essential tie to maintaining the relationship. This was why, in this particular study, adherence was so high. Van de Straten et al. (2012) and Gupta et al. (2013) both highlighted the importance of adherence in explaining the

varied effectiveness (the intent to treat) of the various studies carried out. That is, while they were clearly biologically efficacious (in dramatically reducing transmission and acquisition), in real life, not all participants were able to use drugs as regularly as prescribed.

10. Van Damme et al. 2012.

11. See http://aids.about.com/od/hivmedicationfactsheets/a/drugcost.htm for current costs of individual AIDS medications (often taken in combination with other drugs).

12. Herper 2009, 2012.

13. D'Adesky 2006; Nolen 2007; Barnard 2002; Frontline 2006.

14. www.gilead.com/news/press-releases/2004/7/gilead-reduces-price-of-viread-in-the-developing-world-by-37-percent-antihiv-medication-available-to-68-resourcelimited-countries-through-the-gilead-access-program.

15. To give an illustration, table A5 in the appendix provides very crude estimates of these costs if we decided to focus on an early test-and-treat program for just young women, assuming we could encourage them to adhere to the treatment. The program would aim to conduct HIV testing among young women, and provide ARV treatment in early therapy to all those who are infected in order to reduce their likelihood of transmitting it to their partners. The table shows young women's HIV-prevalence rates in a sample of East and Southern African countries, estimates the population size of young women in those age groups, the size of the HIV positive population, and the cost of providing each infected young woman with ARV medication for a year at $1 a day. Even at dramatically reduced prices—for example, 50 cents a day or 25 cents a day, these amounts are still substantial, and most of the cost would be borne by international donors. These estimates are for one year; these costs would have to be sustained for the next 20–30 years of their lives.

16. UNAIDS 2012.

17. Eaton et al. 2012; Nosyk and Montaner 2012; Meyer-Rath and Over 2012.

18. Creese et al. 2002; Marseille et al. 2002; Canning 2006.

19. McKinlay and McKinlay 1977; Freund and McGuire 1999.

20. Green et al. 2002; Stoneburner and Low-Beer 2004; Kirby 2008; Green 2003; Green and Ruark 2011. The latter go on to argue for interventions focusing on Primary Behavior Change (PBC)—Abstinence and Partner Reduction—rather than technologies such as condom use and HIV testing. See also Halperin et al. 2011 and for Zimbabwe where, even though age at sexual debut remained the same, they argue declines were driven by men's reduction of extramarital partners (who they could no longer afford because of economic decline in the country) and increased condom use with nonmarital partners.

21. Green et al. 2002.

22. Campbell et al. 2005; Blankenship et al. 2006; Dworkin and Ehrhardt 2007; Auerbach, Parkhurst, and Cáceres 2011.

# Bibliography

Abimiku, Alash'le, and Robert C. Gallo. 1995. "HIV: Basic Virology and Pathophysiology." In *HIV Infection in Women,* edited by Howard Minkoff, Jack A. DeHovitz, and Ann Duerr, 13–32. New York: Raven Press.

Acheson, James M. 1981. "Anthropology of Fishing." *Annual Review of Anthropology* 10:275–316.

Agesa, Jacqueline, and Richard U. Agesa. 2002. "Gender Differences in Public and Private University Enrollment in Kenya: What Do They Mask?" *Review of Black Political Economy,* Summer.

Agnew, Robert. 1994. *Delinquency and the Desire for Money. Justice Quarterly* 11 (3): 411–27.

Agot, Kawango E., Ann Vander Stoep, Melissa Tracy, Billy A. Obare, Elizabeth A. Bukusi, Jeckoniah O. Ndinya-Achola, Stephen Moses, and Noel S. Weiss. 2010. "Widow Inheritance and HIV Prevalence in Bondo District, Kenya: Baseline Results from a Prospective Cohort Study." *PLoS ONE* 5 (11): e14028. doi:10.1371/journal.pone.0014028.

Ahlberg, Beth Maina. 1994. "Is There a Distinct African Sexuality? A Critical Response to Caldwell et al." *Africa-London-International African Institute* 64:220–42.

Al-Samarrai, Samer, and Paul Bennell. 2007. "Where Has All the Education Gone in Sub-Saharan Africa? Employment and Other Outcomes among Secondary School and University Leavers." *Journal of Development Studies* 43 (7): 1270–300.

Ankomah, Augustine. 1996. "Premarital Relationships and Livelihoods in Ghana." *Focus on Gender* 4 (3): 39–47.

———. 1999. *Sex, Love, Money and AIDS: The Dynamics of Premarital Sexual Relationships in Ghana. Sexualities* 2 (3): 291–308.

Arbache, Jorge Sabaa, Alexandre Kolev, and Ewa Filipiak. 2010. *Gender Disparities in Africa's Labor Market.* Washington, DC: World Bank Publications.

Arnold, Guy. 1981. *Modern Kenya.* London: Longman.

Ashforth, Adam. 1999. "Weighing Manhood in Soweto." *Codesria Bulletin* 3–4:51–58.

Atieno Odhiambo, Eisha S. 2001. "Kula Raha: Gendered Discourses and the Contours of Leisure in Nairobi, 1946–63." *Azania: Archaeological Research in Africa* 36–37:1, 254–64.

Auerbach, Judith D., Justin O. Parkhurst, and Carlos F. Cáceres. 2011. "Addressing Social Drivers of HIV/AIDS for the Long-Term Response: Conceptual and Methodological Considerations." *Global Public Health*: 1–17.

Auvert, Bertran, Anne Buve, Emmanuel Lagarde, M. Kahindo, J. Chege, N. Rutenberg, R. Musonda, M. Laourou, E. Akam, and H.A. Weiss for the Study Group on the Heterogeneity on HIV Epidemics in African Cities. 2001. "Male Circumcision and HIV Infection in Four Cities in Sub-Saharan Africa." *AIDS* 15, supplement 4:S31–S40.

Auvert, B., D. Taljaard, E. Lagarde, J. Sobngwi-Tambekou, R. Sitta, A. Puren. 2005. "Randomized, Controlled Intervention Trial of Male Circumcision for Reduction of HIV Infection Risk: The ANRS 1265 Trial." *PLoS Med* 2:1–11.

Ayikukwei, R., D. Ngare, J. Sidle, D. Ayuku, J. Baliddawa, and J. Greene. 2008. "HIV/AIDS and Cultural Practices in Western Kenya: The Impact of Sexual Cleansing Rituals on Sexual Behaviors." *Culture, Health and Sexuality* 10 (6): 587–99.

Baeten, J.M., D. Donnell, P. Ndase, N.R. Mugo, J.D. Campbell, J. Wangisi, J.W. Tappero, E.A. Bukusi, C.R. Cohen, E. Katabira, A. Ronald, E. Tumwesigye, E. Were, K.H. Fife, J. Kiarie, C. Farquhar, G. John-Stewart, A. Kakia, J. Odoyo, A. Mucunguzi, E. Nakku-Joloba, R. Twesigye, K. Ngure, C. Apaka, H. Tamooh, F. Gabona, A. Mujugira, D. Panteleeff, K.K. Thomas, L. Kidoguchi, M. Krows, J. Revall, S. Morrison, H. Haugen, M. Emmanuel-Ogier, L. Ondrejcek, R.W. Coombs, L. Frenkel, C. Hendrix, N.N. Bumpus, D. Bangsberg, J.E. Haberer, W.S. Stevens, J.R. Lingappa, and C. Celum for the Partners PrEP Study Team. 2012. "Antiretroviral Prophylaxis for HIV Prevention in Heterosexual Men and Women." *New England Journal of Medicine* 367 (5): 399–410.

Bailey, Beth. 1989. *From Front Porch to Back Seat: Courtship in Twentieth-Century America.* Baltimore: Johns Hopkins University Press.

Bailey, R. C., R. Muga, R. Poulussen, and H. Abicht. 2002. "The Acceptability of Male Circumcision to Reduce HIV Infections in Nyanza Province, Kenya, AIDS Care." *Psychological and Socio-Medical Aspects of AIDS/HIV* 14:1, 27–40.

Bailey, Robert C., Stephen Moses, Corette B. Parker, Kawango Agot, Ian Maclean, John N. Krieger, Carolyn F. M. Williams, Richard T. Campbell, and Jeckoniah O. Ndinya-Achola. 2007. "Male Circumcision for HIV Prevention in Young Men in Kisumu, Kenya: A Randomized Controlled Trial." *Lancet* 369:643–56.

Baird, Sarah, Craig McIntosh, and Berk Özler. 2011. "Cash or Condition? Evidence from a Cash Transfer Experiment." *Quarterly Journal of Economics* 126:1709–753.

Baird, Sarah, Ephraim Chirwa, Craig McIntosh and Berk Özler. 2010. "The Short-Term Impacts of a Schooling Conditional Cash Transfer Program on the Sexual Behavior of Young Women." *Health Economics* 19, supplement 1:55–68.

Baird, Sarah J., Richard S. Garfein, Craig T. McIntosh, Berk Özler. 2012. "Effect of a Cash Transfer Programme for Schooling on Prevalence of HIV and Herpes Simplex Type 2 in Malawi: A Custer Randomised Trial." *Lancet* 379:1320–29.

Baker, Wayne E., and Jason B. Jimerson. 1992. "The Sociology of Money." *American Behavioral Scientist* 35 (6): 678–93.

Bankole, Akinrinola, Susheela Singh, Rubina Hussain, and Gabrielle Oestreicher. 2009. "Condom Use for Preventing STI/HIV and Unintended Pregnancy among Young Men in Sub-Saharan Africa." *American Journal of Men's Health* 3 (1): 60–78.

Barnard, David. 2002. "In the High Court of South Africa, Case No. 4138/98: The Global Politics of Access to Low-Cost AIDS Drugs in Poor Countries." *Kennedy Institute of Ethics Journal* 12 (2): 159–74.

Barnett, Tony, and Alan Whiteside. 2002. *AIDS in the 21st Century: Disease and Globalization.* London: Routledge.

Bearman, Peter S., James Moody, and Katherine Stovel. 2004. "Chains of Affection: The Structure of Adolescent Romantic and Sexual Networks." *American Journal of Sociology* 110 (1): 44–91.

Béné, Christophe, and Sonja Merten. 2008. "Women and Fish-for-Sex: Transactional Sex, HIV/AIDS and Gender in African Fisheries." *World Development* 36 (5): 875–99.

Bennell, Paul. 2003. "The AIDS Epidemic in Sub-Saharan Africa: Are Teachers a High-Risk Group?" *Comparative Education* 39 (4): 493–508.

———. 2005. "The Impact of the AIDS Epidemic on the Schooling of Orphans and Other Directly Affected Children in Sub-Saharan Africa." *Journal of Development Studies* 41 (3): 467–88.

Beoku-Betts, Josephine A. 1998. "Gender and Formal Education in Africa: An Exploration of the Opportunity Structure at the Secondary and Tertiary Levels." In *Women and Education in Sub-Saharan Africa: Power, Opportunities and Constraints*, edited by Marianne Bloch, Josephine A. Beoku-Betts, and B. Robert Tabachnick, 157–84. Boulder: Lynne Rienner.

Bernstein, Elizabeth. 2010. *Temporarily Yours: Intimacy, Authenticity, and the Commerce of Sex*. Chicago: University of Chicago Press.

Bicego, George, Shea Rutstein, and Kiersten Johnson. 2003. "Dimensions of the Emerging Orphan Crisis in Sub-Saharan Africa." *Social Science and Medicine* 56:1235–47.

Bingenheimer, Jeffrey B. 2007. "Wealth, Wealth Indices and HIV Risk in East Africa." *International Family Planning Perspectives* 33 (2): 83–84.

Blankenship, Kim, Sam Friedman, Shari Dworkin, and J. E. Mantell. 2006. "Structural Interventions: Concepts, Challenges and Opportunities for Research." *Journal of Urban Health: Bulletin of the New York Academy of Medicine* 83 (1): 59–72.

Bledsoe, Caroline. 1990. *School Fees and the Marriage Process for Mende Girls in Sierra Leone*. In *Beyond the Second Sex: New Directions in the Anthropology of Gender*, edited by Peggy Reeves Sanday and Ruth Gallagher Goodenough, 283–309. Philadelphia: University of Pennsylvania Press.

Bledsoe, Caroline H., John B. Casterline, Jennifer A. Johnson-Kuhn, and John G. Haaga, eds. 1998. *Critical Perspectives on Schooling and Fertility in the Developing World*. Washington, DC: National Academy Press.

Bloch, Maurice, and Jonathan Parry. 1989. "Introduction: Money and the Morality of Exchange." In *Money and the Morality of Exchange*, edited by Jonathan Parry and Maurice Bloch, 1–32. New York: Cambridge University Press.

Blount, Ben G. 1973. "Luo of South Nyanza, Western Kenya." In *Cultural Source Materials for Population Planning in East Africa*, vol. 3, *Beliefs and Practices*, edited by Angela Molnos, 318–29. Nairobi: Institute of African Studies, University of Nairobi, Ford Foundation.

Boerma, J. Ties, and Sharon S. Weir. 2005. "Integrating Demographic and Epidemiological Approaches to Research on HIV/AIDS: The Proximate-Determinants Framework." *Journal of Infectious Diseases* 191, supplement 1:S61–67.

Bogle, Kathleen. 2008. *Hooking Up: Sex, Dating and Relationships on Campus*. New York: New York University Press.

Bogonko, Sorobea Nyachico. 1992. *A History of Modern Education in Kenya, 1895–1991*. London: Evans Brothers (Kenya).

Boily, Marie-Claude, Rebecca F. Baggaley, Lei Wang, Benoit Masse, Richard G. White, Richard J. Hayes, and Michel Alary. 2009. "Heterosexual Risk of HIV-1 Infection per Sexual Act: Systematic Review and Meta-Analysis of Observational Studies." *Lancet Infectious Diseases* 9:118–29.

Bolan, Gail, Anke A. Ehrhardt, and Judith N. Wasserheit. 1999. "Gender Perspectives and STDs." In *Sexually Transmitted Diseases*, 3rd ed., edited by King K. Holmes, Per-Anders Mardh, P. Frederick Sparling, Stanley M. Lemon, Walter E. Stamm, Peter Piot, and Judith N. Wasserheit, 117–28. New York: McGraw-Hill Professional.

Bold, Tessa, Mwangi Kimenyi, Germano Mwabu, and Justin Sandefur. 2013. "Why Did Abolishing Fees Not Increase Public School Enrollment in Kenya?" *Africa Growth Initiative. Brookings Institute.* Working Paper 4, January 2013.

Booth, Karen M. 2003. *Local Women, Global Science: Fighting AIDS in Kenya.* Bloomington: Indiana University Press.

Bouvet, E., I. De Vincenzi, R. Ancelle, and F. Vachon. 1989. "Defloration as Risk Factor for Heterosexual HIV Transmission." *Lancet* 1:615.

Bradshaw, York. 1993. "State Limitations, Self-Help Secondary Schooling and Development in Kenya." *Social Forces* 72 (2): 347–78.

Branch, Daniel. 2011. *Kenya: Between Hope and Despair, 1963–2011.* New Haven: Yale University Press.

Brenner, Suzanne. 1998. "Gender and the Domestication of Desire." In *The Domestication of Desire: Women, Wealth and Modernity in Java*, edited by Suzanne Anne Brenner, 134–70. Princeton, NJ: Princeton University Press.

Brint, Steven. 2006. *Schools and Societies.* 2nd ed. Stanford: Stanford University Press.

Brown, B. Bradford. 1990. "Peer Groups and Peer Cultures." In *At the Threshold: The Developing Adolescent*, edited by S. Shirley Feldman and Glen R. Elliott, 171–96. Cambridge, MA: Harvard University Press.

Bryceson, Deborah Fahy. 2002. "Multiplex Livelihoods in Rural Africa: Recasting the Terms and Conditions of Gainful Employment." *Journal of Modern African Studies* 40 (1): 1–28.

Buchmann, Claudia. 1999. "The State and Schooling in Kenya: Historical Developments and Current Challenges." *Africa Today* 46 (1): 94–117.

Budig, Michelle J., and Paula England. 2001. "The Wage Penalty for Motherhood." *American Sociological Review* 66 (2): 204–25.

Bureau of Labor Statistics. 2013. Highlights of Women's Earnings in 2012. *Bureau of Labor Statistics Reports.* October 2013: Report 1045.

Burke, Timothy. 1996. *Lifebuoy Men, Lux Women: Commodification, Consumption and Cleanliness in Modern Zimbabwe.* Durham: Duke University Press.

Buvé, A., M. Carael, R.J. Hayes, B. Auvert, B. Ferry, N.J. Robinson, S. Anagonou, L. Kanhonou, M. Laouro, and S. Abega. 2001. "The Multicentre Study on Factors Determining the Differential Spread of HIV in Four African Cities: Summary and Conclusions." *AIDS* 15, supplement 4:S127–S31.

Caldwell, John. 1980. "Mass Education as a Determinant of the Timing of Fertility Decline." *Population and Development Review* 6 (2): 225–55.

Caldwell, John C., and Pat Caldwell. 1993. "The Nature and Limits of the Sub-Saharan African AIDS Epidemic: Evidence from Geographic and Other Patterns." *Population and Development Review* 19 (4): 817–48.

Caldwell, John, Pat Caldwell, and Pat Quiggin. 1989. "The Social Context of AIDS in Africa." *Population and Development Review* 15 (2): 185–234.

Cameron, D. William, Lourdes J. D'Costa, Gregory M. Maitha, Mary Cheang, Peter Piot, Francis A. Plummer, J. Neil Simonsen, Allan R. Ronald, Michael N. Gakinya, J. O. Ndinya-Achola, and Robert C. Brunham. 1989. "Female to Male Transmission of Human Immunodeficiency Virus Type 1: Risk Factors for Seroconversion in Men." *Lancet* 8660:403–7.

Camlin, Carol S., Zachary A. Kwena, and Shari L. Dworkin. 2013. "Jaboya vs. Jakambi: Status, Negotiation, and HIV Risks among Female Migrants in the 'Sex for Fish' Economy in Nyanza Province, Kenya." *AIDS Education and Prevention* 25 (3): 216–31.

Campbell, Catherine. 1997. "Migrancy, Masculine Identities and AIDS: The Psychosocial Context of HIV Transmission on the South African Gold Mines." *Social Science and Medicine* 45 (2): 273–81.

———. 2003. *"Letting Them Die": Why HIV/AIDS Intervention Programmes Fail.* Bloomington: Indiana University Press.

Campbell, C., A. Foulis, S. Maimane, and Z. Sibiya. 2005. "The Impact of Social Environments on the Effectiveness of Youth HIV Prevention: A South African Case Study." *AIDS Care: Psychological and Socio-Medical Aspects of AIDS/HIV* 17 (4): 471–78.

Canagarajah, Sudharshan, and Helena Skyt Nielsen. 2001. "Child Labor in Africa: A Comparative Study." *Annals of the American Academy of Political and Social Science* 575:71–91.

Canning, David. 2006. "The Economics of HIV/AIDS in Low-Income Countries: The Case for Prevention." *Journal of Economic Perspectives* 20 (3): 121–42.

Carruthers, Bruce G., and Wendy Nelson Espeland. 1998. "Money, Meaning and Morality." *American Behavioral Scientist* 41 (10): 1384–408.

Carsten, Janet. 1989. "Cooking Money: Gender and the Symbolic Transformation of Means of Exchange in a Malay Fishing Community." In *Money and the Morality of Exchange,* edited by Jonathan Parry and Maurice Bloch, 116–41. New York: Cambridge University Press.

Carswell, J. Wilson, Graham Lloyd, and Julian Howells. 1989. "Prevalence of HIV-1 in East African Lorry Drivers." *AIDS* 3:759–61.

Carter, Anthony T. 1999. "What Is Meant and Measured by 'Education'?" In *Critical Perspectives on Schooling and Fertility in the Developing World,* edited by Caroline H. Bledsoe, John B. Casterline, Jennifer A. Johnson-

Kuhn, and John G. Haaga, 49–79. Washington, DC: National Academy Press.

Chan, Selina. 2006. "Love and Jewelry: Patriarchal Control, Conjugal Ties and Changing Identities." In *Modern Loves: The Anthropology of Romantic Courtship and Companionate Marriage,* edited by Jennifer Hirsch and Holly Wardlow, 35–50. Ann Arbor: University of Michigan Press.

Chant, Sylvia, and Gareth A. Jones. 2005. "Youth, Gender and Livelihoods in West Africa: Perspectives from Ghana and The Gambia." *Children's Geographies* 3 (2): 185–99.

Charles, Maria. 1992. "Cross-National Variation in Occupational Sex Segregation." *American Sociological Review* 57:483–502.

Charles, Maria, and Karen Bradley. 2009. "Indulging Our Gendered Selves? Sex Segregation by Field of Study in 44 Countries." *American Journal of Sociology* 114 (4): 924–76.

Charmaz, Kathy. 2001. "Grounded Theory." In *Contemporary Field Research: Perspectives and Formulations,* edited by Robert Emerson, 335–52. Prospect Heights: Waveland Press.

Chatterji, Minki, Nancy Murray, David London, and Philip Anglewicz. 2004. *The Factors Influencing Transactional Sex Among Young Men and Women in 12 Sub-Saharan African Countries.* USAID: Policy Project.

Chemaitelly, Hiam, and Laith J. Abu-Raddad. 2013. "External Infections Contribute Minimally to HIV Incidence among HIV Sero-Discordant Couples in Sub-Saharan Africa." *Sexually Transmitted Infections* 89:138–41.

Cherlin, Andrew J. 2009. *The Marriage-Go-Round: The State of Marriage and the Family in America Today.* New York: Vintage.

Chu, Jessica. 2011. "Gender and 'Land Grabbing' in Sub-Saharan Africa: Women's Land Rights and Customary Land Tenure." *Development* 54 (1): 35–39.

Clark, Shelley. 2004. "Early Marriage and HIV Risks in Sub-Saharan Africa." *Studies in Family Planning* 35 (3): 149–60.

Clark, Shelley, Caroline Kabiru, and Rohini Mathur. 2010. "Relationship Transitions among Youth in Urban Kenya." *Journal of Marriage and Family* 72:73–88.

Cleland, John, Mohamed M. Ali, Iqbal Shah. 2006. "Trends in Protective Behaviour among Single vs. Married Young Women in Sub-Saharan Africa: The Big Picture." *Reproductive Health Matters* 14 (28): 17–22.

Cohen, David William, and E. S. Atieno Odhiambo. 1989. *Siaya: The Historical Anthropology of an African Landscape.* London: James Currey.

Cohen, Myron S. M. D., Ying Q. Chen, PhD, Marybeth McCauley, MPH, Theresa Gamble, PhD, Mina C. Hosseinipour, MD, Nagalingeswaran Kumarasamy, MB, BS, James G. Hakim, MD, Johnstone Kumwenda, FRCP, Beatriz Grinsztejn, MD, Jose H. S. Pilotto, MD, Sheela V. Godbole, MD, Sanjay

Mehendale, MD, Suwat Chariyalertsak, MD, Breno R. Santos, MD, Kenneth H. Mayer, MD, Irving F. Hoffman, PA, Susan H. Eshleman, MD, Estelle Piwowar-Manning, MT, Lei Wang, PhD, Joseph Makhema, FRCP, Lisa A. Mills, MD, Guy de Bruyn, MB, BCh, Ian Sanne, MB, BCh, Joseph Eron, MD, Joel Gallant, MD, Diane Havlir, MD, Susan Swindells, MB, BS, Heather Ribaudo, PhD, Vanessa Elharrar, MD, David Burns, MD, Taha E. Taha, MB, BS, Karin Nielsen-Saines, MD, David Celentano, ScD, Max Essex, DVM, and Thomas R. Fleming, PhD, for the HPTN 052 Study Team. 2011. "Prevention of HIV-1 Infection with Early Antiretroviral Therapy." *New England Journal of Medicine* 365:493–505.

Colclough, Christopher, and Andrew Webb. 2012. "A Triumph of Hope over Reason? Aid Accords and Education Policy in Kenya. *Comparative Education* 48 (2): 263–80.

Cole, Jennifer. 2004. "Fresh Contact in Tamatave, Madagascar: Sex, Money, and Intergenerational Transformation." *American Ethnologist* 31 (4): 573–88.

———. 2005. "The Jaombilo of Tamatave (Madagascar), 1992–2004: Reflections on Youth and Globalization." *Journal of Social History*, Summer.

———. 2010. *Sex and Salvation: Imagining the Future in Madagascar.* Chicago: University of Chicago Press.

Cole, Jennifer, and Deborah Durham. 2007. "Introduction: Age, Regeneration, and the Intimate Politics of Globalization." In *Generations and Globalization: Youth, Age and the Family in the New World Economy*, edited by Jennifer Cole and Deborah Durham. Bloomington: Indiana University Press.

Comaroff, Jean, and John L. Comaroff. 2000. *Millenial Capitalism: First Thoughts on a Second Coming. Public Culture* 12 (2): 291–343.

———. 2006. "Beasts, Banknotes and the Colour of Money in Colonial South Africa." *Archaeological Dialogues* 12 (2): 107–32.

———. 2012. "Theory from the South: Or, How Euro-America Is Evolving Toward Africa." *Anthropological Forum: A Journal of Social Anthropology and Comparative Sociology* 22 (2): 113–31.

Coontz, Stephanie. 2005. *Marriage, a History: How Love Conquered Marriage.* New York: Penguin.

Cornwall, Andrea. 2002. "Spending Power: Love, Money and the Reconfiguration of Gender Relations in Ado-Odo, Southwestern Nigeria." *American Ethnologist* 29 (4): 963–80.

Creese, Andrew, Katherine Floyd, Anita Alban, Lorna Guinness. 2002. "Cost-Effectiveness of HIV/AIDS Interventions in Africa: A Systematic Review of the Evidence." *Lancet* 359: 1635–42.

D'Adesky, Anne-Christine. 2006. *Moving Mountains: The Race to Treat Global AIDS.* New York: Verso.

Daley, Elizabeth, and Birgit Englert. 2010. "Securing Land Rights for Women." *Journal of Eastern African Studies* 4 (1): 91–113.

Day, Lynda R. 1998. "Rites and Reason: Precolonial Education and Its Relevance to the Current Production and Transmission of Knowledge." In *Women and Education in Sub-Saharan Africa: Power, Opportunities and Constraints,* edited by Marianne Bloch, Josephine A. Beoku-Betts, and B. Robert Tabachnick, 49–72. Boulder: Lynne Rienner.

de Walque, Damien. 2007. "Sero-Discordant Couples in Five African Countries: Implications for Prevention Strategies." *Population and Development Review* 33 (3): 501–23.

de Walque, Damien, Jessica S. Nakiyingi-Miiro, June Busingye, and Jimmy A. Whitworth. 2005. "Changing Association between Schooling Levels and HIV-1 Infection over 11 Years in a Rural Population Cohort in South-West Uganda." *Tropical Medicine and International Health* 10 (10): 993–1001.

Dore, Robert. 1976. *The Diploma Disease: Education, Qualification and Development.* Berkeley: University of California Press.

Dude, Annie M. 2007. *Intimate Partner Violence and HIV Risk in Kenya.* Unpublished manuscript.

Duflo, Esther, Pascaline Dupas, Michael Kremer, and Samuel Sinei. 2006. "Education and HIV/AIDS Prevention: Evidence from a randomized evaluation in Western Kenya." *World Bank Policy Research Working Paper* 4024, October 2006.

Dunbar, Megan S., M. Catherine Maternowska, Mi-Suk J. Kang, Susan M. Laver, Imelda Mudekunye-Mahaka, and Nancy S. Padian. 2010. "Findings from SHAZ!: A Feasibility Study of a Microcredit and Life-Skills HIV Prevention Intervention to Reduce Risk Among Adolescent Female Orphans in Zimbabwe." *Journal of Prevention & Intervention in the Community* 38 (2): 147–61.

Dunkle, Kristin L., Rachel K. Jewkes, Heather C. Brown, Glenda E. Gray, James A. McIntryre, and Siobán D. Harlow. 2004. "Transactional Sex among Women in Soweto, South Africa: Prevalence, Risk Factors, and Association with HIV Infection." *Social Science and Medicine* 59:1581–92.

Dupas, Pascaline. 2011. "Do Teenagers Respond to HIV Risk Information? Evidence from a Field Experiment in Kenya." *American Economic Journal: Applied Economics* 3:1–34.

DuPré, Carole E. 1968. *The Luo of Kenya: An Annotated Bibliography.* Washington, DC: Institute for Cross Cultural Research.

Dworkin, Shari L., and Anke A. Ehrhardt. 2007. "Going Beyond 'ABC' to Include 'GEM': Critical Reflections on Progress in the HIV/AIDS Epidemic." *American Journal of Public Health* 97:13–18.

Dworkin, Shari L., and Kim Blankenship. 2009. "Microfinance and HIV/AIDS Prevention: Assessing Its Promise and Limitations." *AIDS & Behavior* 13:462–69.

Dworkin, Shari L., Shelly Grabe, Tiffany Lu, Abbey Hatcher, Zachary Kwena, Elizabeth Bukusi, and Esther Mwaura-Muiru. 2012. "Property Rights Violations as a Structural Driver of Women's HIV Risks: A Qualitative Study in Nyanza and Western Provinces, Kenya." *Archives of Sexual Behavior,* 42(5):703–713.

Eaton, Jeffrey W., Leigh F. Johnson, Joshua A. Salomon, Till Bärnighausen, Eran Bendavid, Anna Bershteyn, David E. Bloom et al. 2012. "HIV Treatment as Prevention: Systematic Comparison of Mathematical Models of the Potential Impact of Antiretroviral Therapy on HIV Incidence in South Africa." *PLoS medicine* 9 (7): e1001245.

Eckholm, Peter. 1977. *The Picture of Health: Environmental Sources of Disease.* New York: W. W. Norton.

Eisemon, Thomas Owen, and John Schwille. 1991. "Primary Schooling in Burundi and Kenya: Preparation for Secondary Education or for Self-Employment?" *Elementary School Journal* 92 (1): 23–39.

Eisenstein, Hester. 2009. *Feminism Seduced: How Global Elites Use Women's Labor and Ideas to Exploit the World.* Boulder: Paradigm Publishers.

Eloundou-Enyegue, Parfait M., and Julie Davanzo. 2003. "Economic Downturns and Schooling Inequality, Cameroon, 1987–95." *Population Studies* 57 (2): 183–97.

Emerson, Robert M., Rachel I. Fretz, and Linda L. Shaw. 1995. *Writing Ethnographic Fieldnotes.* Chicago: University of Chicago Press.

England, Paula, Emily Fitzgibbons Shafer, and Alison C. K. Fogarty. 2007. "Hooking Up and Forming Romantic Relationships on Today's College Campuses." In *The Gendered Society Reader,* edited by Michael Kimmel and Amy Aronson, 578–91. New York: Oxford University Press, 2011.

Epstein, Edward J. 1982. "Have You Ever Tried to Sell a Diamond?" *Atlantic Monthly,* February.

Epstein, Helen. 2007. *The Invisible Cure: Africa, the West, and the Fight against AIDS.* New York: Farrar, Straus and Giroux.

Erulkar, Annabel, Judith Bruce, Aleke Dondo, Jennefer Sebstad, James Matheka, Arjmand Banu Khan, and Ann Gathuku. 2006. "Tap and Reposition Youth (TRY): Providing Social Support, Savings and Microcredit Opportunities for Young Women in Areas with High HIV Prevalence." *Seeds* 23.

Evans, David, Michael Kremer, and Mũthoni Ngatia. 2009. "The Impact of Distributing School Uniforms on Children's Education in Kenya." *Poverty Action Lab.*

Evans-Pritchard, E. E. 1935. "Witchcraft." *Africa: Journal of the International African Institute* 8 (4): 417–22.

———. 1950. "Marriage Customs of the Luo of Kenya." In The *Position of Women in Primitive Societies, and Other Essays in Social Anthropology,* 228–44. London: Faber and Faber, 1965.

Eyawo, Oghenowede, Damien de Walque, Nathan Ford, Gloria Gakii, Richard T. Lester, Edward J. Mills. 2010. "HIV Status in Discordant Couples in Sub-Saharan Africa: A Systematic Review and Meta-Analysis." *Lancet Infectious Diseases* 10:770–77.

Fearn, Hugh. 1961. *An African Economy: A Study of the Economic Development of the Nyanza Province of Kenya, 1903–1953.* East African Institute of Social Research by Oxford University Press.

Fenton, Kevin A., Anne M. Johnson, Sally McManus, and Bob Erens. 2001. "Measuring Sexual Behavior: Methodological Challenges in Survey Research." *Sexually Transmitted Infections* 77:84–92.

Ferguson, James. 1992. "The Cultural Topography of Wealth: Commodity Paths and the Structure of Property in Rural Lesotho." *American Anthropologist* 94 (1): 55–73.

———. 1994. *The Anti-Politics Machine: "Development," Depoliticization, and Bureaucratic Power in Lesotho.* New York: Cambridge University Press.

———. 1999. *Expectations of Modernity: Myths and Meanings of Urban Life on the Zambian Copperbelt.* California: University of California Press.

———. 2006. *Global Shadows: Africa in the Neoliberal World Order.* Durham: Duke University Press.

Fine, Michelle. 1988. "Sexuality, Schooling & and Adolescent Females: The Missing Discourse of Desire." *Harvard Educational Review* 58 (1): 29–53.

Fleming, D. T., and J. N. Wasserheit. 1999. "From Epidemiological Synergy to Public Health Policy and Practice: The Contribution of Other Sexually Transmitted Diseases to Sexual Transmission of HIV Infection." *Sexually Transmitted Infections* 75:3–17.

Flood, Michael. 2003. "Lust, Trust And Latex: Why Young Heterosexual Men Do Not Use Condoms." *Culture, Health & Sexuality* 5 (4): 353–69.

Fortson, Jane. 2008. "The Gradient in Sub-Saharan Africa: Socioeconomic Status and HIV/AIDS." *Demography* 45 (2): 303–22.

Fox, Ashley M. 2010. "The Social Determinants of HIV Serostatus in Sub-Saharan Africa: An Inverse Relationship between Poverty and HIV?" *Public Health Reports* 125, supplement 4:16–24.

———. 2012. "The HIV-Poverty Thesis Re-Examined: Poverty, Wealth or Inequality as a Social Determinant of HIV Infection in Sub-Saharan Africa." *Journal of Biosocial Science* 44 (4): 459–80.

Freund, Peter E. S., and Meredith B. McGuire. 1999. *Health, Illness and the Social Body: A Critical Sociology.* 3rd ed. New Jersey: Prentice Hall.

Friedman, Andrea. 2001. "Book Reviews: The Politics of Consumption: Women and Consumer Culture." *Journal of Women's History* 13 (2): 159–68.

Frontline. 2006. "The Age of AIDS." Public Broadcasting Service. www.pbs.org /wgbh/pages/frontline/aids/.

Frye, Margaret. 2012. "Bright Futures in Malawi's New Dawn: Educational Aspirations as Assertions of Identity." *American Journal of Sociology* 117 (6): 1565–624.

Fuller, Bruce. 1991. *Growing-Up Modern: The Western State Builds Third-World Schools*. New York: Routledge.

Furstenberg, Frank F. 2000. "The Sociology of Adolescence and Youth in the 1990s: A Critical Commentary." *Journal of Marriage and the Family* 62:896–910.

Gargano, Julia W., Kayla Laserson, Hellen Muttai, Frank Odhiambo, Vincent Orimba, Mirabelle Adamu-zeh, John Williamson, Maquins Sewe, Lennah Nyabiage, Karen Owuor, Dita Broza, Barbara Marston, and Marta Ackers. 2012. "The Adult Population Impact of HIV Care and Antiretroviral Therapy (ART)—Nyanza Province, Kenya, 2003–2008." *AIDS* 26:1–10.

Geheb, Kim, and Tony Binns. 1997. "'Fishing Farmers' or 'Farming Fishermen'? The Quest for Household Income and Nutritional Security on the Kenyan Shores of Lake Victoria." *African Affairs* 96 (382): 73–93.

Geissler, Wenzel, and Ruth Jane Prince. 2010. *The Land Is Dying: Contingency, Creativity and Conflict in Western Kenya*. Vol. 5. New York: Berghahn.

Glenn, Norval, and Elizabeth Marquardt. 2001. *Hooking Up, Hanging Out and Hoping for Mr. Right: College Women on Dating and Mating Today*. An Institute for American Values Report to the Independent Women's Forum.

Glick, Peter J., and David E. Sahn. 2008. "Are Africans Practicing Safer Sex? Evidence from Demographic and Health Surveys for Eight Countries." *Economic Development and Cultural Change* 56:397–439.

Glynn, Judith R., Michel Caraël, Anne Buve, Séverin Anagonou, Léopold Zekeng, Maina Kahindo, and Rosemary Musonda for the Study Group on Heterogeneity of HIV Epidemics in African Cities. 2004. "Does Increased General Schooling Protect against HIV Infection? A Study in Four African Cities." *Tropical Medicine and International Health* 9 (1): 4–14.

Glynn, Judith R., Michel Caraël, Betran Auvert, Maina Kahindo, Jane Chege, Rosemary Musonda, Frederick Kaona, and Anne Buvé. 2001. "Why Do Young Women Have a Much Higher Prevalence of HIV Than Young Men? A Study in Kisumu, Kenya and Ndola, Zambia." *AIDS* 15 (2001): S51–S60.

Gouws, Eleanor, Karen A. Stanecki, Rob Lyerla, and Peter D. Ghys. 2008. "The Epidemiology of HIV Infection among Young People Aged 15–24 Years in Southern Africa." *AIDS* 22, supplement 4:S5–S16.

Grant, Robert M., Javier R. Lama, Peter L. Anderson, Vanessa McMahan, Albert Y. Liu, Lorena Vargas, Pedro Goicochea, Martín Casapía, Juan Vicente Guanira-Carranza, Maria E. Ramirez-Cardich, Orlando Montoya-Herrera, Telmo Fernández, Valdilea G. Veloso, Susan P. Buchbinder, Suwat Chariyalertsak, Mauro Schechter, Linda-Gail Bekker, Kenneth H. Mayer, Esper Georges Kallás, K. Rivet Amico, Kathleen Mulligan, Lane R.

Bushman, Robert J. Hance, Carmela Ganoza, Patricia Defechereux, Brian Postle, Furong Wang, J. Jeff McConnell, Jia-Hua Zheng, Jeanny Lee, James F. Rooney, Howard S. Jaffe, Ana I. Martinez, David N. Burns, and David V. Glidden for the iPrEx Study Team. 2010. "Preexposure Chemoprophylaxis for HIV Prevention." In Men Who Have Sex with Men, *New England Journal of Medicine* 363 (27): 2587-99.

Gray, Ronald H., Godfrey Kigozi, David Serwadda, Frederick Makumbi, Stephen Watya, Fred Nalugoda, Noah Kiwanuka, Lawrence H. Moulton, Mohammad A. Chaudhary, Michael Z. Chen, Nelson K. Sewankambo, Fred Wabwire-Mangen, Melanie C. Bacon, Carolyn F. M. Williams, Pius Opendi, Steven J. Reynolds, Oliver Laeyendecker, Thomas C. Quinn, and Maria J. Wawer. 2007. "Male Circumcision for HIV Prevention in Men in Rakai, Uganda: A Randomised Trial." *Lancet* 369:657-66.

Gray, Ronald H., Maria J. Wawer, Ron Brookmeyer, Nelson K. Sewankambo, David Serwadda, Fre Wabwire-Mangen, Tom Lutalo, Xianbin Li, Thomas van Cott, Thomas C. Quinn, and the Rakai Project Team. 2001. "Probability of HIV-1 Transmission per Coital Act in Monogamous, Heterosexual, HIV-1-Discordant Couples in Rakai, Uganda." *Lancet* 357:1149-53.

Green, Edward Crocker. 2003. *Rethinking AIDS Prevention: Learning from Successes in Developing Countries.* Greenwood.

Green, Edward C., and Allison Herling Ruark. 2011. *AIDS, Behavior and Culture: Understanding Evidence Based Prevention.* Walnut Creek, CA: Left Coast Press.

Green, Edward, Vinand Nantulya, Rand Stoneburner, and John Stover. 2002. *What Happened in Uganda? Declining HIV Prevalence, Behavior Change and the National Response.* Edited by Janice A. Hogle. Washington, DC: USAID.

Gregson, Simon, Constance A. Nyamukapa, Geoffrey P. Garnett, Peter R. Mason, Tom Zhuwau, Michel Caräel, Stephen K. Chandiwana, and Roy M. Anderson. 2002. "Sexual Mixing Patterns and Sex-Differentials in Teenage Exposure to HIV Infection in Rural Zimbabwe." *Lancet* 359 (9321): 1896-903.

Gregson, Simon, Heather Waddell, and Stephen Chandiwana. 2001. "School Education and HIV Control in Sub-Saharan Africa: From Discord to Harmony?" *Journal of International Development* 13 (4): 467-85.

Griffin, Christine. 2004. "Good Girls, Bad Girls: Anglocentrism and Diversity in the Constitution of Contemporary Girlhood." In *All about the Girl: Culture, Power and Identity,* edited by Anita Harris, 29-43. New York: Routledge.

Gupta, Neeru, and Mary Mahy. 2003. "Sexual Initiation among Adolescent Girls and Boys: Trends and Differentials in Sub-Saharan Africa." *Archives of Sexual Behavior* 32 (1): 41-53.

Gupta, Ravindra K., Mark A. Wainberg, Francoise Brun-Vezinet, Jose M. Gatell, Jan Albert, Anders Sönnerborg, and Jean B. Nachega. 2013. "Oral

Antiretroviral Drugs as Public Health Tools for HIV Prevention: Global Implications for Adherence, Drug Resistance, and the Success of HIV Treatment Programs." *Journal of Infectious Diseases* 207, supplement 2:S101–S106.

Guyer, Jane I. 1994. "Lineal Identities and Lateral Networks: The Logic of Polyandrous Motherhood." In *Nuptiality in Sub-Saharan Africa: Contemporary Anthropological and Demographic Perspectives,* edited by Caroline Bledsoe and Gilles Pison, 231–52. Oxford: Clarendon Press.

Halperin, Daniel T., and Helen Epstein. 2004. "Concurrent Sexual Partnerships Help to Explain Africa's High HIV Prevalence: Implications for Prevention." *Lancet* 364 (9428): 4–5.

Halperin, Daniel T., Owen Mugurungi, Timothy B. Hallett, Backson Muchini, Bruce Campbell, Tapuwa Magure, Clemens Benedikt, and Simon Gregson. 2011. "A Surprising Prevention Success: Why Did the HIV Epidemic Decline in Zimbabwe?" *PLoS Medicine* 8 (2): 1–7.

Hamilton, Laura, and Elizabeth A. Armstrong. 2009. "Gendered Sexuality in Young Adulthood: Double Binds and Flawed Options." *Gender & Society* 23 (5): 589–616.

Hansen, Karen Tranberg. 1999. "Second-Hand Clothing Encounters in Zambia: Global Discourses, Western Commodities, and Local Histories." *Africa: Journal of the International African Institute* 69 (3): 343–65.

Haram, Liv. 1995. "Negotiating Sexuality in Times of Economic Want: The Young and Modern Meru Women." In *Young People at Risk: Fighting AIDS in Northern Tanzania,* edited by Knut-Inge Klepp, Paul M. Biswalo, and Aud Talle, 31–48. Oslo: Scandinavian University Press.

Hargreaves, James R., Christopher P. Bonell, Tania Boler, Delia Boccia, Isolde Birdthistle, Adam Fletcher, Paul M. Pronyk, and Judith R. Glynn. 2008. "Systematic Review Exploring Time Trends in the Association between Educational Attainment and Risk of HIV Infection in Sub-Saharan Africa." *AIDS* 22:403–14.

Harris, Anita. 2004. "Jamming Girl Culture: Young Women and Consumer Citizenship." In *All about the Girl: Culture, Power, and Identity,* edited by Anita Harris, 163–72. New York: Routledge.

Harrison, Abigail. 2008. "Hidden Love: Sexual Ideologies and Relationship Ideals among Rural South African Adolescents in the Context of HIV/AIDS." *Culture, Health & Sexuality* 10 (2): 175–89.

Hay, Margaret Jean. 1976. "Luo Women and Economic Change during the Colonial Period." In *Women in Africa: Studies in Social and Economic Change,* edited by Nancy J. Hafkin and Edna G. Bay, 87–109. Stanford: Stanford University Press.

Heald, Suzette. 1995. "The Power of Sex: Some Reflections on the Caldwells' 'African Sexuality' Thesis." *Africa: Journal of the African Institute* 65 (4): 489–505.

Helleringer, Stéphane, and Hans-Peter Kohler. 2007. "Sexual Network Structure and the Spread of HIV in Africa: Evidence from Likoma Island, Malawi." *AIDS* 21:2323–32.

Herper, Matthew. 2009. "The Profit Pill." *Forbes,* March 23. www.forbes.com/2009/03/23/hiv-aids-gilead-business-health-care-viread.html.

———. 2012. "The Truly Staggering Cost of Inventing New Drugs." *Forbes,* February 10. www.forbes.com/sites/matthewherper/2012/02/10/the-truly-staggering-cost-of-inventing-new-drugs.

Hewett, Paul, Barbara S. Mensch, and Annabel S. Erulkar. 2004. "Consistency in the Reporting of Sexual Behavior by Adolescent Girls in Kenya: A Comparison of Interviewing Methods." *Sexually Transmitted Infections* 80, supplement 2:S43–S48.

Higgins, Jenny A., Susie Hoffman, and Shari L. Dworkin. 2010. "Rethinking Gender, Heterosexual Men, and Women's Vulnerability to HIV/AIDS." *American Journal of Public Health* 100 (3): 435–45.

Hill Collins, Patricia. 2004. *Black Sexual Politics: African Americans, Gender and the New Racism.* New York: Routledge.

Hirsch, Jennifer, and Holly Wardlow, eds. 2006. *Modern Loves: The Anthropology of Romantic Courtship and Companionate Marriage.* Ann Arbor: University of Michigan Press.

Hirsch, Jennifer S., Holly Wardlow, Daniel Jordan Smith, Harriet M. Phinney, Shanti Parikh, and Constance A. Nathanson. 2009. *The Secret: Love, Marriage and HIV.* Nashville: Vanderbilt University Press.

Hirsch, Jennifer S., Jennifer Higgins, Margaret E. Bentley, and Constance A. Nathanson. 2002. "The Social Constructions of Sexuality: Marital Infidelity and Sexually Transmitted Disease—HIV Risk in a Mexican Migrant Community." *American Journal of Public Health* 92 (8): 1227–37.

Hitchcock, P., and L. Fransen. 1999. "Preventing HIV Infection: Lessons from Mwanza and Rakai." *Lancet* 9152:513.

Hodges, Melissa J., and Michelle J. Budig. 2010. "Who Gets the Daddy Bonus?: Organizational Hegemonic Masculinity and the Impact of Fatherhood on Earnings." *Gender & Society* 24 (6): 717–45.

Hogan, Dennis P., and Nan Marie Astone. 1986. "The Transition to Adulthood." *Annual Review of Sociology* 12:109–30.

Hornsby, Charles. 2012. *Kenya: A History since Independence.* New York: IB Tauris.

Hughes, Rees. 1994. "Legitimation, Higher Education and the Post-Colonial State: A Comparative Study of India and Kenya." *Comparative Education* 30 (3): 193–204.

Hugonnet, Stéphane, Frank Mosha, James Todd, Kokugonza Mugeye, Arnoud Klokke, Leonard Ndeki, David Ross, Heiner Grosskurth, and Richard Hayes. 2002. "Incidence of HIV Infection in Stable Sexual Partnerships: A

Retrospective Cohort Study of 1802 Couples in Mwanza Region, Tanzania." *Journal of Acquired Immune Deficiency Syndromes* 30 (1): 73–80.

Hunter, Lori M., Roger-Mark De Souza, and Wayne Twine. 2008. "The Environmental Dimensions of the HIV/AIDS Pandemic: A Call for Scholarship and Evidence-Based Intervention." *Population and Environment* 29 (3): 103–7.

Hunter, Mark. 2002. The Materiality of Everyday Sex: Thinking beyond 'Prostitution.'" *African Studies* 61 (1): 99–120.

———. 2010. *Love in the Time of AIDS: Intimacy, Gender and Rights in South Africa*. Bloomington: Indiana University Press.

Iliffe, John. 2006. *The African AIDS Epidemic: A History*. Oxford: James Currey.

Ilouz, Eva. 1997. *Consuming the Romantic Utopia: Love and the Cultural Contradictions of Capitalism*. Berkeley: University of California Press.

Jejheeboy, Shireen J. 1995. *Women's Education, Autonomy and Reproductive Behavior: Experience from Developing Countries*. Oxford: Clarendon Press.

Jessor, Richard. 1991. "Risk Behavior in Adolescence: A Psychosocial Framework for Understanding and Action." *Journal of Adolescent Health* 12 (8): 597–605.

Johnson-Hanks, Jennifer. 2002. "On the Limits of Life Stages in Ethnography: Toward a Theory of Vital Conjunctures." *American Anthropologist* 104 (3): 865–80.

———. 2006. *Uncertain Honor: Modern Motherhood in an African Crisis*. Chicago: University of Chicago Press.

Jukes, Matthew, Stephanie Simmons, and Donald Bundy. 2008. "Education and Vulnerability: the Role of Schools in Protecting Young Women and Girls from HIV in Southern Africa." *AIDS* 22, supplement 4:S41–S56.

Kabiru, Caroline W., Nancy Luke, Chimaraoke O. Izugbara, and Eliya M. Zulu. 2010. "The Correlates of HIV Testing and Impacts on Sexual Behavior: Evidence from a Life History Study of Young People in Kisumu, Kenya." *BMC Public Health* 10:412.

Kabiru, Caroline W., Sanyu A. Mojola, Donatien Beguy, and Chinelo Okigbo. 2013. "Growing Up at the 'Margins': Concerns, Aspirations and Expectations of Young People Living in Nairobi's Slums." *Journal of Research on Adolescence Special Issue: Adolescents in the Majority World* 23(1): 81–94.

Kakooza, James, and Sitawa R. Kimuna. 2005. "HIV/AIDS Orphans' Education in Uganda: The Changing Role of Older People." *Journal of Intergenerational Relationships* 3 (4): 63–81.

Kakubo-Mariara, Jane, and Domisiano K. Mwabu. 2007. "Determinants of School Enrolment and Education Attainment: Empirical Evidence from Kenya." *South African Journal of Economics* 75 (3): 572–93.

Kaler, Amy. 2001. "Many Divorces and Many Spinsters: Marriage as an Invented Tradition in Southern Malawi, 1946–1999." *Journal of Family History* 26 (4): 529–56.

Karanja, Wambui wa. 1994. "The Phenomenon of 'Outside Wives': Some Reflections on Its Possible Influence on Fertility." In *Nuptiality in Sub-Saharan Africa: Contemporary Anthropological and Demographic Perspectives*, edited by Caroline Bledsoe and Gilles Pison, 194–214. Oxford: Clarendon Press.

Kateregga, Eseza, and Thomas Sterner. 2009. "Lake Victoria Fish Stocks and the Effects of Water Hyacinth." *Journal of Environment and Development* 18 (1): 62–78.

Kaufman, Carol E., and Stavros E. Stavrou. 2004. "'Bus Fare Please': The Economics of Sex and Gifts among Young People in Urban South Africa." *Culture, Health and Sexuality* 6 (5): 377–91.

Kearns, Robin A. 1993. "Place and Health: Towards a Reformed Medical Geography." *Professional Geographer* 45 (2): 139–47.

Keister, Lisa A. 2002. "Financial Markets, Money and Banking." *Annual Review of Sociology* 28:39–61.

Kelly, Michael J. 2000. "Standing Education on Its Head: Aspects of Schooling in a World with HIV/AIDS." *Current Issues in Comparative Education* 3 (1): 28–38.

Kenya, Republic of. *District Development Plans, Bondo, Nyando, Kisumu and Homa Bay*. Nairobi: Rural Planning Department, Office of the Vice President and Ministry of Planning and National Development.

*Kenya Demographic and Health Survey* (KDHS). 1989. Calverton, MD: National/Central Bureau of Statistics (Kenya); Ministry of Health (Kenya); and ORC/ICF Macro.

*Kenya Demographic and Health Survey* (KDHS). 1993. Calverton, MD: National/Central Bureau of Statistics (Kenya); Ministry of Health (Kenya); and ORC/ICF Macro.

*Kenya Demographic and Health Survey* (KDHS). 1999. Calverton, MD: National/Central Bureau of Statistics (Kenya); Ministry of Health (Kenya); and ORC/ICF Macro.

*Kenya Demographic and Health Survey* (KDHS). 2004. Calverton, MD: National/Central Bureau of Statistics (Kenya); Ministry of Health (Kenya); and ORC/ICF Macro.

*Kenya Demographic and Health Survey* (KDHS). 2010. Calverton, MD: National/Central Bureau of Statistics (Kenya); Ministry of Health (Kenya); and ORC/ICF Macro.

Kenya Education Directory. 2006. Nairobi: Express Communications.

Kim, Julia, Paul Pronyk, Tony Barnett, and Charlotte Watts. 2008. "Exploring the Role of Economic Empowerment in HIV Prevention." *AIDS* 22, supplement 4:S57–S71.

Kiragu, K., M. Kimani, C. Manathoko, and C. Mackenzie. 2006. *Teachers Matter: Baseline Findings on HIV-Related Needs of Kenyan Teachers*. Horizons Research Update. Washington, DC: Population Council.

Kirby, Douglas. 2008. "Changes in Sexual Behaviour Leading to the Decline in the Prevalence of HIV in Uganda: Confirmation from Multiple Sources of Evidence." *Sexually Transmitted Infections* 84, supplement 2:S35–S41.

Komba-Malekela, Betty, and Rita Liljeström. 1994. "Looking for Men." In *Chelewa, Chelewa: The Dilemma of Teenage Girls,* edited by Zubeida Tumbo-Masabo and Rita Liljeström, 133–49. Nordiska Africainstitutet: Scandinavian Institute of African Studies.

Konde-Lule, Joseph K., N. Sewankambo, and Martina Morris. 1997. "Adolescent Sexual Networking and HIV Transmission in Rural Uganda." *Health Transition Review* 7, supplement: 89–100.

Kretschmar, M., and M. Morris. 1995. "Concurrent Partnerships and Transmission Dynamics in Networks." *Social Networks* 17:299–318.

Kwena, Zachary A., Elizabeth Bukusi, Enos Omondi, Musa Ng'ayo, and King K. Holmes. 2012. "Transactional Sex in the Fishing Communities along Lake Victoria, Kenya: A Catalyst for the Spread of HIV." *African Journal of AIDS Research* 11:1, 9–15.

Laga, Marie, Bernhard Schwärtlander, Elisabeth Pisani, Papa Salif Sow, and Michel Caraël. 2001. "To Stem HIV in Africa, Prevent Transmission to Young Women." *AIDS* 15:931–34.

Laumann, Edward O., John H. Gagnon, Robert T. Michael, and Stuart Michaels. 1994. *The Social Organization of Sexuality: Sexual Practices in the United States.* Chicago: University of Chicago Press.

Leach, Fiona, Vivian Fiscian, Esme Kadzamira, Eve Lemani, and Pamela Machakanja. 2003. *An Investigative Study into the Abuse of Girls in African Schools.* DFID Education Research 54. London: Department for International Development.

Leclerc-Madlala, Suzanne. 2002. "Youth, HIV/AIDS and the Importance of Sexual Culture and Context." *Social Dynamics* 28 (1): 20–41.

———. 2003. "Transactional Sex and the Pursuit of Modernity." *Social Dynamics* 29 (2): 213–33.

———. 2008. "Age-Disparate and Intergenerational Sex in Southern Africa: The Dynamics of Hypervulnerability." *AIDS* 22:S17–S25.

Lelei, Macrina. 2005. "Girls' Education in Kenya: Problems and Prospects in Global Context." In *African Women and Globalization: Dawn of the 21st Century,* edited by Jepkorir Rose Chepyator-Thomson, 153–81. Trenton, NJ: Africa World Press.

Lelei, Macrina C., and John C. Weidman. 2012. "Education Development in Kenya: Enhancing Access and Quality." In *Quality and Qualities: Tensions in Education Reforms,* edited by Clementina Acedo, Don Adams, and Simona Popa, 143–62. Rotterdam: Sense Publishers.

Lloyd, Cynthia B., ed. 2005. *Growing Up Global: The Changing Transitions to Adulthood in Developing Countries.* Panel on Transitions to Adulthood in

Developing Countries. Committee on Population and Board on Children, Youth, and Families. Division of Behavioral and Social Sciences and Education. Washington, DC: National Academics Press.

Lloyd, Cynthia B., Carol E. Kaufman, and Paul Hewett. 2000. "The Spread of Primary Schooling in Sub-Saharan Africa: Implications for Fertility Change." *Population and Development Review* 26 (3): 483–515.

Longfield, Kim, Anne Glick, Margaret Waithaka, and John Berman. 2004. "Relationships between Older Men and Younger Women: Implications for STIs/HIV in Kenya." *Studies in Family Planning* 35 (2): 125–34.

Luke, Nancy. 2003. "Age and Economic Asymmetries in the Sexual Relationships of Adolescent Girls in Sub-Saharan Africa." *Studies in Family Planning* 34 (2): 67–86.

———. 2005. "Confronting the 'Sugar Daddy' Stereotype: Age and Economic Asymmetries and Risky Sexual Behavior in Urban Kenya." *International Family Planning Perspectives* 31 (1): 6–14.

———. 2006. "Exchange and Condom Use in Informal Sexual Relationships in Urban Kenya." *Economic Development and Cultural Change* 54 (2): 319–48.

———. 2010. "Migrants' Competing Commitments: Sexual Partners in Urban Africa and Remittances to the Rural Origin." *American Journal of Sociology* 115 (5): 1435–79.

Luke, Nancy, and Kathleen Kurz. 2002. *Cross-Generational and Transactional Sexual Relations in Sub-Saharan Africa: Prevalence of Behavior and Implications for Negotiating Safer Sex Practices.* Washington, DC: International Center for Research on Women.

Luke, Nancy, Rachel E. Goldberg, Blessing U. Mberu, and Eliya M. Zulu. 2011. "Social Exchange and Sexual Behavior in Young Women's Premarital Relationships in Kenya." *Journal of Marriage and Family* 73:1048–64.

Lurie, Mark N., Brian G. Williams, Khangelani Zuma, David Mkaya-Mwamburi, Geoff P. Garnett, Adriaan W. Sturm, Michael D. Sweat, Joel Gittelsohn, and Salim S. Abdool Karim. 2003a. "The Impact of Migration on HIV-1 Transmission in South Africa: A Study of Migrant and Nonmigrant Men and Their Partners." *Sexually Transmitted Diseases* 30 (2): 149–56.

Lurie, Mark N., Brian G. Williams, Khangelani Zuma, David Mkaya-Mwamburi, Geoff P. Garnett, Michael D. Sweat, Joel Gittelsohn, and Salim S. Abdool Karim. 2003b. "Who Infects Whom? HIV-1 Concordance and Discordance among Migrant and Non-Migrant Couples in South Africa." *AIDS* 17:2245–52.

Macintyre, Sally, and Anne Ellaway. 2000. "Ecological Approaches: Rediscovering the Role of the Physical and Social Environment." In *Social Epidemiology*, edited by Lisa F. Berkman and Ichiro Kawachi, 332–48. New York: Oxford University Press.

MacPhail, Catherine, and Catherine Campbell. 2001. "'I Think Condoms Are Good but, Aai, I Hate Those Things': Condom Use among Adolescents and Young People in a Southern African Township." *Social Science and Medicine* 52:1613–27.

Maharaj, Pranitha, and John Cleland. 2005. "Risk Perception and Condom Use Among Married or Cohabiting Couples in KwaZulu-Natal, South Africa." *International Family Planning Perspectives* 31 (1): 24–29.

Mail and Guardian. 2007. "Kenya Calls for Action to Save Receding Lake Victoria." *Mail and Guardian,* June 11.

*Malawi Demographic and Health Survey 2004.* MDHS. 2005. Calverton, MD: National Statistical Office (Malawi) and ORC Macro.

*Malawi Demographic and Health Survey 2010.* MDHS. 2005. Calverton, MD: National Statistical Office (Malawi) and ORC Macro.

Malo, Shadrack. 1999. *Luo Customs and Practices.* Nairobi: ScienceTech Network.

Marseille, Elliot, Paul B. Hofmann, and James G. Kahn. 2002. "HIV Prevention before HAART in Sub-Saharan Africa." *Lancet* 359 (9320): 1851–56.

Mastro, Timothy D., Glen A. Satten, Taweesak Nopkesorn, Suebpong Sangkharomya, and Ira M. Longini, Jr. 1994. "Probability of Female to Male Transmission of HIV-1 in Thailand." *Lancet* 343 (8891): 204–7.

Maurer, Bill. 2006. "The Anthropology of Money." *Annual Review of Anthropology* 35:15–36.

Mauss, Marcel. 1990. *The Gift: The Form and Reason for Exchange in Archaic Societies.* Translated by W. D. Halls. New York: W. W. Norton.

Mbembé, J. A., and Sarah Nuttall. 2004. "Writing the World from an African Metropolis." *Public Culture* 16 (3): 347–72.

Mboya, Paul, and Jane Achieng. 2001. *Paul Mboya's "Luo Kitgi Gi Timbegi": A Translation into English.* Nairobi: Atai.

Mboya, Tom M. 2012. "The Serious People of Raha: The Politics in the Ethnic Stereotyping of the Luo in Okatch Biggy's Benga." In *Rethinking Eastern African Literary and Intellectual Landscapes,* edited by James Ogude, Grace A. Musila, and Dina Ligaga, 263–82. Trenton, NJ: Africa World Press.

Mbugua, G. G., L. N. Muthami, C. W. Mutura, S. A. Oogo, P. G. Waiyaki, C. P. Lindan, and N. Hearst. 1995. "Epidemiology of HIV Infection among Long Distance Truck Drivers in Kenya." *East African Medical Journal* 72 (8): 515–18.

Mbugua, Njeri. 2007. "Factors Inhibiting Educated Mothers in Kenya from Giving Meaningful Sex-Education to Their Daughters." *Social Science and Medicine* 64:1079–89.

McGowan, Abigail. 2006. "An All Consuming Subject? Women and Consumption in Late-Nineteenth and Early Twentieth Century Western India." *Journal of Women's History* 18 (4): 31–54.

McKinlay, John B., and Sonja M. McKinlay. 1977. "The Questionable Contribution of Medical Measures to the Decline of Mortality in the United States in the Twentieth Century." *Milbank Memorial Fund Quarterly. Health and Society*: 405–28.

McNeely, Clea A., and Brian K. Barber. 2010. "How Do Parents Make Adolescents Feel Loved? Perspectives on Supportive Parenting from Adolescents in 12 Cultures." *Journal of Adolescent Research* 25 (4): 601–31.

McRobbie, Angela. 1997. "Bridging the Gap: Feminism, Fashion and Consumption." *Feminist Review* 55:73–89.

MDG Center Nairobi Environmental Team and Millenium Cities Initiative. 2009. "An Overview of the Main Environmental Issues Affecting Kisumu and Lake Victoria's Winam Gulf." *MCI Social Sector Working Paper Series* No 02/2009. Earth Institute, Columbia University.

Meekers, Dominique, and Anne-Emmanuèle Calvès. 1997. "'Main' Girlfriends, Girlfriends, Marriage, and Money: The Social Context of HIV Risk Behavior in Sub-Saharan Africa." *Health Transition Review* 7, supplement: 361–75.

Mensch, Barbara S., and Cynthia B. Lloyd. 2001. "Gender Differences in the Schooling Experiences of Adolescents in Low-Income Countries: The Case of Kenya." *Studies in Family Planning* 29 (2): 167–84.

Mensch, Barbara S., Judith Bruce, and Margaret E. Greene. 1998. *The Uncharted Passage: Girls' Adolescence in the Developing World*. New York: Population Council.

Merten, Sonja, and Tobias Haller. 2007. "Culture, Changing Livelihoods, and HIV/AIDS Discourse: Reframing the Institutionalization of Fish-for-Sex Exchange in the Zambian Kafue Flats." *Culture, Health & Sexuality* 9 (1): 69–83.

Merton, Robert K. 1968. "Social Structure and Anomie." In *Social Theory and Social Structure*, 185–214. New York: Free Press.

Meyer-Rath, Gesine, and Mead Over. 2012. "HIV Treatment as Prevention: Modelling the Cost of Antiretroviral Treatment—State of the Art and Future Directions." *PLoS Medicine* 9 (7): e1001247.

Mills, David, and Richard Ssewakiryanga. 2005. "No Romance without Finance: Commodities, Masculinities and Relationships among Kampalan Students." In *Readings in Gender in Africa*, edited by Andrea Cornwall, 90–94. Bloomington: Indiana University Press.

Mishra, Vinod, and Simona Bignami-Van Assche. 2008. "Orphans and Vulnerable Children in High HIV-Prevalence Countries in Sub-Saharan Africa." DHS Analytical Studies 15. Calverton, MD: Macro International.

Mishra, Vinod, Simona Bignami-Van Assche, Robert Greener, Martin Vaessen, Rathavuth Hong, Peter D. Ghys, J. Ties Boerma, Ari Van Assche, Shane Khan, and Shea Rutstein. 2007. "HIV Infection Does Not Disproportionately Affect the Poorer in Sub-Saharan Africa." *AIDS* 21, supplement 7:S17–S28.

Mojola, Sanyu A. 2011a. "Fishing in Dangerous Waters: Ecology, Gender and Economy in HIV Risk." *Social Science and Medicine* 72 (2): 149–56.

———. 2011b. "Multiple Transitions and HIV Risk among Orphaned Kenyan School Girls." *Studies in Family Planning* 42 (1): 29–40.

———. 2014. "Providing Women, Kept Men: Doing Masculinity in the Wake of the African HIV/AIDS Pandemic." *Signs* 39 (2): 341–63.

Mojola, Sanyu A., and Bethany Everett. 2012. "STD and HIV Risk Factors among U.S. Young Adults: Variations by Gender, Race, Ethnicity and Sexual Orientation." *Perspectives in Sexual and Reproductive Health* 44 (2): 125–33.

Moore, Ann M., Ann E. Biddlecom, and Eliya M. Zulu. 2007. "Prevalence and Meanings of Exchange of Money or Gifts for Sex in Unmarried Adolescent Sexual Relationships in Sub-Saharan Africa." *African Journal of Reproductive Health* 11 (3): 44–61.

Morris, Martina, Chai Podhisita, Maria J. Wawer, and Mark S. Handcock. 1996. "Bridge Populations in the Spread of HIV/AIDS in Thailand." *AIDS* 10 (11): 1265–71.

Muriungi, Agnes. 2005. "'Chira': The (Re-)Construction of Moral Economies in Contemporary Kenya." In *Romance, Love and Gender in Times of Crisis: HIV/AIDS in Kenyan Popular Fiction*, 172–204. PhD Diss., University of Witswatersrand.

Muya, Wamahiu. 2000. "The Vital Role of Education in Kenya's Economy." *Daily Nation*, March 6.

Muyanga, Milu, John Olwande, Esther Mueni, and Stella Wambugu. 2010. "Free Primary Education in Kenya: An Impact Evaluation Using Propensity Score Methods." In *Child Welfare in Developing Countries*, 125–55. New York: Springer.

Mwiria, Kilemi. 1990. "Kenya's Harambee Secondary School Movement: The Contradictions of Public Policy." *Comparative Education Review* 34 (3): 350–68.

———. 1991. "Education for Subordination: African Education in Colonial Kenya." *History of Education* 20 (3): 261–73.

Negin, Joel, James Wariero, Robert G. Cumming, Patrick Mutuo, and Paul M. Pronyk. 2010. "High Rates of AIDS-Related Mortality among Older Adults in Rural Kenya." *JAIDS: Journal of Acquired Immune Deficiency Syndromes* 55 (2): 239–44.

Ngau, Peter M. 1987. "Tensions in Empowerment: The Experience of the 'Harambee' (Self-Help) Movement in Kenya." *Economic Development and Cultural Change* 35 (3): 523–38.

Ngware, Moses W., Eldah N. Onsomu, David I. Muthaka, and Damiano K. Manda. 2006. "Improving Access to Secondary Education in Kenya: What Can Be Done?" *Equal Opportunities International* 25 (7): 523–43.

Nishimura, Mikiko, and Takashi Yamano. 2012. "Emerging Private Education in Africa: Determinants of School Choice in Rural Kenya." *World Development* 43:266–75.

Njiru, M., J. Kazungu, C. C. Ngugi, J. Gichuki, and L. Muhoozi. 2008. "An Overview of the Current Status of Lake Victoria Fishery: Opportunities, Challenges and Management Strategies." *Lakes & Reservoirs: Research and Management* 13:1–12.

Njiru, M., P. Nzungi, A. Getabu, E. Wakwabi, A. Othina, T. Jembe, and S. Wekesa. 2006. "Are Fisheries Management Measures in Lake Victoria Successful? The Case of Nile Perch and Nile Tilapia Fishery." *African Journal of Ecology* 45:315–23.

Njue, Carolyne, Helene A. C. M. Voeten, and Pieter Remes. 2009. "Disco Funerals: A Risk Situation for HIV Infection among Youth in Kisumu, Kenya." *AIDS* 23:505–9.

Nnko, Soori, J. T. J. Ties Boerma, Mark Urassa, Gabriel Mwaluko, and Basia Zaba. 2004. "Secretive Females or Swaggering Males: An Assessment of the Quality of Sexual Partnership Reporting in Rural Tanzania." *Social Science and Medicine* 59 (2): 299–310.

Nolen, Stephanie. 2007. *28 Stories of AIDS in Africa*. London: Portobello Books.

Nosyk, Bohdan, and Julio S. G. Montaner. 2012. "The Evolving Landscape of the Economics of HIV Treatment and Prevention." *PLoS Medicine* 9 (2): e1001174.

Nyambedha, Erick Otieno, Simiyu Wandibba, and Jens Aagaard-Hansen. 2003. "Changing Patterns of Orphan Care due to the HIV Epidemic in Western Kenya." *Social Science & Medicine* 57 (2): 301–11.

Nyamnjoh, Francis B. 2005. "Fishing in Troubled Waters: Disquettes and Thiofs in Dakar." *Africa* 75 (3): 295–323.

Nyanzi, Stella, Barbara Nyanzi, Bessie Kalina, and Robert Pool. 2004. "Mobility, Sexual Networks and Exchange among Bodabodamen in Southwest Uganda." *Culture, Health and Sexuality* 6 (3): 239–54.

Nzomo, Maria. 1989. "The Impact of the Women's Decade on Policies, Programs and Empowerment of Women in Kenya." *Issue: A Journal of Opinion* 17 (2): 9–17.

Ochieng, William R. 1979. *People around the Lake—Luo*. London: Evans Brothers.

Ocholla-Ayayo, A. B. C. 1977. *The Luo Culture: A Reconstruction of the Material Culture Patterns of a Traditional African Society*. Wiesbaden: Steiner.

———. 1997. "HIV/AIDS Risk Factors and Changing Sexual Practices in Kenya." In *African Families and the Crisis of Social Change*, edited by Thomas S. Weisner, Candice Bradley, and Philip Leroy Kilbride, 109–24. Westport, CT: Greenwood.

Odada, Eric O., Washington O. Ochola, and Dan O. Olago. 2009. "Drivers of Ecosystem Change and Their Impacts on Human Well-Being in Lake Victoria Basin." *African Journal of Ecology* 47, supplement 1:46–54.

Odinga, Oginga. 1967. *Not Yet Uhuru*. London: Heinemann.

O'Farrell, Nigel. 2001. "Enhanced Efficiency of Female to Male Transmission in Core Groups in Developing Countries: The Need to Target Men." *Sexually Transmitted Diseases* 28 (2): 84–91.

Ogot, Bethwell A. 2004. *Politics and the AIDS Epidemic in Kenya, 1983–2003*. Kisumu, Kenya: Anyange Press.

———. 2009. *A History of the Luo-Speaking Peoples of Eastern Africa*. Kisumu, Kenya: Anyange Press.

Okeyo, T. M., and A. K. Allen. 1994. "Influence of Widow Inheritance on the Epidemiology of AIDS in Africa." *African Journal of Medical Practice* 1 (1): 20–25.

Okoko, Tervil. 2000. "Scientists Move to Save Lake Victoria From Dying." *Panafrican News Agency*. Allafrica.com.

Ominde, Simeon Hongo. 1987. *The Luo Girl: From Infancy to Marriage*. Nairobi: Kenya Literature Bureau.

Omolo, Jacob. 2012. "Youth Employment in Kenya: Analysis of Labour Market and Policy Interventions." *FES Kenya Occasional Paper* 1:1–24.

Ong'or, Basil Tito, and Shu Long-Cang. 2007. "Water Supply Crisis and Mitigation Options in Kisumu City, Kenya." *Water Resources Development* 23 (3): 485–500.

ORC Macro International. www.measuredhs.com.

O'Rourke, Meghan. 2007. "Diamonds Are a Girl's Worst Friend: The Trouble with Engagement Rings." *Slate*, June 11.

Oruboloye, I. O., John C. Caldwell, and Pat Caldwell. 1993. "The Role of High Risk Occupations in the Spread of AIDS: Truck Drivers and Itinerant Market Women in Nigeria." *International Family Planning Perspectives* 19:43–48.

Osler, Audrey. 1993. "Education for Development and Democracy in Kenya: A Case Study." *Educational Review* 45 (2): 165–73.

Padian, Nancy S., Sandra I. McCoy, Salim S. Abdool Karim, Nina Hasen, Julia Kim, Michael Bartos, Elly Katabira, Stefano M. Bertozzi, Bernhard Schwartländer, and Myron S. Cohen. 2011. "HIV Prevention Transformed: The New Prevention Research Agenda." *Lancet* 378 (9787): 269–78.

Padian, Nancy S., Stephen C. Shiboski, Sarah O. Glass, and Eric Vittinghoff. 1997. "Heterosexual Transmission of Human Immunodeficiency Virus (HIV) in Northern California: Results from a Ten-Year Study." *American Journal of Epidemiology* 146 (4): 350–57.

Parkhurst, Justin O. 2010. "Understanding the Correlations between Wealth, Poverty and Human Immunodeficiency Virus Infection in African Countries." *Bulletin of the World Health Organization* 88:519–26.

Parkin, David. 1978. *The Cultural Definition of Political Response: Lineal Destiny among the Luo*. London: Academic Press.

Parry, Jonathan, and Maurice Bloch, eds. 1989. *Money and the Morality of Exchange*. New York: Cambridge University Press.

Paterson, Mark. 2006. *Consumption and Everyday Life*. London: Routledge.

Pepin, Jacques. 2011. *The Origins of AIDS*. New York: Cambridge University Press.

Pettifor, Audrey E., Brooke A. Levandowski, Catherine MacPhail, Nancy S. Padian, Myron S. Cohen, and Helen V. Rees. 2008. "Keep Them in School: The Importance of Education as a Protective Factor against HIV Infection among Young South African Women." *International Journal of Epidemiology* 37 (6): 1266–73.

Pettifor, Audrey, Helen V. Rees, Immo Kleinschmidt, Annie E. Steffenson, Catherine MacPhail, Lindiwe Hlongwa-Madikizela, Kerry Vermaak, and Nancy S. Padian. 2005. "Young People's Sexual Health in South Africa: HIV Prevalence and Sexual Behaviors from a Nationally Representative Household Survey." *AIDS* 19:1525–34.

Pickering, H., M. Okongo, K. Bwanika, B. Nnalusiba, and J. Whitworth. 1997. "Sexual Behavior in a Fishing Community on Lake Victoria, Uganda." *Health Transition Review* 7:13–20.

Population Reference Bureau. 2012. World Population Data Sheet of the Population Reference Bureau. www.prb.org.

Potash, Betty, ed. 1986. *Widows in African Societies: Choices and Constraints*. Stanford: Stanford University Press.

Poulin, Michelle. 2007. "Sex, Money and Premarital Partnerships in Southern Malawi." *Social Science and Medicine* 65:2383–93.

Pronyk, Paul M., James R. Hargreaves, Julia C. Kim, Linda A. Morison, Godfrey Phetla, Charlotte Watts, Joanna Busza, and John D. H. Porter. 2006. "Effect of a Structural Intervention for the Prevention of Intimate-Partner Violence and HIV in Rural South Africa: A Cluster Randomised Trial." *Lancet* 368 (9551): 1973–83.

Pronyk, Paul M., Julia C. Kim, Tanya Abramsky, Godfrey Phetla, James R. Hargreaves, Linda A. Morison, Charlotte Watts, Joanna Busza, and John D. H. Porter. 2008. "A Combined Microfinance and Training Intervention Can Reduce HIV Risk Behaviour in Young Female Participants." *AIDS* 22 (13): 1659–65.

Pugh, Allison J. 2009. *Longing and Belonging: Parents, Children, and Consumer Culture*. Berkeley: University of California Press.

Pyle, Jean L., and Kathryn B. Ward. 2003. "Recasting Our Understanding of Gender and Work during Global Restructuring." *International Sociology* 18 (3): 461–89.

Quinn, Thomas C., Maria J. Wawer, Nelson Sewankambo, David Serwadda, Chuanjun Li, Fred Wabwire-Mangen, Mary O. Meehan, Thomas Lutalo, and Ronald H. Gray. 2000. "Viral Load and Heterosexual Transmission of

Human Immunodeficiency Virus Type 1." *New England Journal of Medicine* 342 (13): 921–29.

Rehle, T. M., T. B. Hallett, O. Shisana, V. Pillay-van Wyk, K. Zuma et al. 2010. "A Decline in New HIV Infections in South Africa: Estimating HIV Incidence from Three National HIV Surveys in 2002, 2005 and 2008." *PLoS ONE* 5 (6): e11094.

Reniers, Georges. 2008. "Marital Strategies for Regulating Exposure to HIV." *Demography* 45 (2): 417–38.

Reniers, Georges, and Rania Tfaily. 2012. "Polygyny, Partnership Concurrency, and HIV Transmission in Sub-Saharan Africa." *Demography* 49 (3): 1075–101.

Reniers, Georges, and Susan Watkins. 2010. "Polygyny and the Spread of HIV in Sub-Saharan Africa: A Case of Benign Concurrency." *AIDS* 24:299–307.

Reskin, Barbara. 1993. "Sex Segregation in the Workplace." *Annual Review of Sociology* 19:241–70.

Reuters. 2011. 2011 Engagement & Jewelry Statistics Released by TheKnot.com & WeddingChannel.com. www.reuters.com/article/2011/08/30/idUS198935+30-Aug-2011+BW20110830.

Reynolds, Heidi W., Winnie K. Luseno, and Ilene S. Speizer. 2012. "The Measurement of Condom Use in Four Countries in East and Southern Africa." *AIDS and Behavior* 16 (4): 1044–53.

Rindfuss, Ronald R. 1991. "The Young Adult Years: Diversity, Structural Change, and Fertility." *Demography* 28 (4): 493–512.

Ross, Catherine E., and Chia-ling Wu. 1995. The Links between Education and Health." *American Sociological Review* 60 (5): 719–45.

Røttingen, John-Arne, D. William Cameron, and Geoffrey P. Garnett. 2001. "A Systematic Review of the Epidemiological Interactions between Classic Sexually Transmitted Diseases and HIV: How Much Really Is Known?" *Sexually Transmitted Diseases* 28 (10): 579–97.

Royce, Rachel A., Arlene Seña, Willard Cates, and Myron S. Cohen. 1997. "Sexual Transmission of HIV. *New England Journal of Medicine* 336 (15): 1072–78.

Rubin, Gayle. 1975. "The Traffic in Women: Notes on the 'Political Economy' of Sex." In *Toward an Anthropology of Women*, edited by Rayna R. Reiter, 157–210. New York: Monthly Review Press.

Ruddick, Sue. 2003. "The Politics of Aging: Globalization and the Restructuring of Youth and Childhood." *Antipode* 35 (2): 334–62.

Schatz, Enid. 2005. "'Take Your Mat and Go!': Rural Malawian Women's Strategies in the HIV/AIDS Era." *Culture, Health & Sexuality* 7 (5): 479–92.

Seeley, Janet A., and Edward H. Allison. 2005. "HIV/AIDS in Fishing Communities: Challenges to Delivering Antiretroviral Therapy to Vulnerable Groups." *AIDS Care* 17 (6): 688–97.

Serpell, Robert. 1993. *The Significance of Schooling: Life Journeys in an African Society*. New York: Cambridge University Press.

Setel, Philip. 1995. AIDS as a Paradox of Manhood and Development in Kilimanjaro, Tanzania." *Social Science and Medicine* 43 (8): 1169–78.

———. 1999. *A Plague of Paradoxes: AIDS, Culture and Demography in Northern Tanzania*. Chicago: University of Chicago Press.

Shanahan, Michael J. 2000. "Pathways to Adulthood in Changing Societies: Variability and Mechanisms in Life Course Perspective." *Annual Review of Sociology* 26:667–92.

Shelton, J. D., M. M. Cassell, J. Adetunji. 2005. "Is Poverty or Wealth at the Root of HIV?" *Lancet* 366:1057–58.

Shipton, Parker M. 1989. *Bitter Money: Cultural Economy and Some African Meanings of Forbidden Commodities*. Washington, DC: American Anthropological Association.

———. 2007. *The Nature of Entrustment: Intimacy, Exchange and the Sacred in Africa*. New Haven: Yale University Press.

Sikoyo, George M., and Lisa Goldman. 2007. "Assessing the Assessments: Case Study of an Emergency Action Plan for the Control of Water Hyacinth in Lake Victoria." *Water Resources Development* 23 (3): 443–55.

Silberschmidt, Margrethe. 1992. "Have Men Become the Weaker Sex? Changing Life Situations in Kisii District, Kenya." *Journal of Modern African Studies* 30 (2): 237–53.

———. 2001. "Disempowerment of Men in Rural and Urban East Africa: Implications for Male Identity and Sexual Behavior." *World Development* 29 (4): 657–71.

———. 2004. "Men, Male Sexuality and HIV/AIDS: Reflections from Studies in Rural and Urban East Africa." *Transformation: Critical Perspectives on Southern Africa* 54 (1): 42–58.

Simmel, Georg. 2004. *The Philosophy of Money*. New York: Routledge.

Smith, Daniel Jordan. 2004. "Premarital Sex, Procreation, and HIV Risk in Nigeria." *Studies in Family Planning* 35 (4): 223–35.

———. 2006. "Love and the Risk of HIV: Courtship, Marriage, and Infidelity in Southeastern Nigeria." In *Modern Loves: The anthropology of romantic courtship and companionate marriage*, edited by Jennifer Hirsch and Holly Wardlow, 135–53. Ann Arbor: University of Michigan Press.

Smith, Kirsten P., and Susan Cotts Watkins. 2005. "Perceptions of Risk and Strategies for Prevention: Responses to HIV/AIDS in Rural Malawi." *Social Science and Medicine* 60:649–60.

Sobek, Matthew Joseph. 1997. "A Century of Work: Gender, Labor Force Participation, and Occupational Attainment in the United States, 1880–1990," PhD diss., University of Minnesota.

Somerset, Anthony. 2011. "Access, Cost and Quality: Tensions in the Development of Primary Education in Kenya." *Journal of Education Policy* 26 (4): 483–97.

Sommer, Marni. 2009. "Ideologies of Sexuality, Menstruation and Risk: Girls' Experiences of Puberty and Schooling in Northern Tanzania." *Culture, Health & Sexuality: An International Journal for Research, Intervention and Care* 11:4, 383–98.

———. 2010. "Where the Education System and Women's Bodies Collide: The Social and Health Impact of Girls' Experiences of Menstruation and Schooling in Tanzania." *Journal of Adolescence* 33 (4): 521–29.

Stambach, Amy. 2000. *Lessons from Mount Kilimanjaro: Schooling, Community and Gender in East Africa.* New York: Routledge.

Steady, Filomina Chioma. 1987. "Polygamy and the Household Economy in a Fishing Village in Sierra Leone." In *Transformations of African Marriage,* edited by David Parkin and David Nyamwaya, 211–29. Manchester: Manchester University Press.

Stewart, Kearsley A. 2001. "Toward a Historical Perspective on Sexuality in Uganda: The Reproductive Lifeline Technique for Grandmothers and Their Daughters." *Africa Today:* 123–48.

Stewart, K., M. Powell, and R. Greer. 2009. "An Alternative to Conventional Sanitary Protection: Would Women Use a Menstrual Cup?" *Journal of Obstetrics & Gynecology* 29 (1): 49–52.

Stirrat, R. L. 1989. "Money, Men and Women." In *Money and the Morality of Exchange,* edited by Jonathan Parry and Maurice Bloch, 94–116. New York: Cambridge University Press.

Stoneburner, Rand L., and Daniel Low-Beer. 2004. "Population-Level HIV Declines and Behavioral Risk Avoidance in Uganda." *Science* 304 (5671): 714–18.

Strauss, Anselm, and Juliet Corbin. 1998. *Basics of Qualitative Research: Techniques and Procedures for Developing Grounded Theory.* 2nd ed. Thousand Oaks, CA: Sage.

Swidler, Ann. 1986. "Culture in Action: Symbols and Strategies." *American Sociological Review* 51 (2): 273–86.

———. 2001. *Talk of Love: How Culture Matters.* Chicago: University of Chicago Press.

Swidler, Ann, and Susan Cotts Watkins. 2007. "Ties of Dependence: AIDS and Transactional Sex in Rural Malawi." *Studies in Family Planning* 38 (3): 147–62.

Tavory, Iddo, and Ann Swidler. 2009. "Condom Semiotics: Meaning and Condom Use in Rural Malawi." *American Sociological Review* 74 (2): 171–89.

Thomas, Lynn. 2008. "The Modern Girl and Racial Respectability in 1930s South Africa." In *The Modern Girl around the World: Consumption,*

*Modernity and Globalization,* edited by Alys Eve Weinbaum, Lynn M. Thomas, Priti Ramamurthy, Uta G. Poiger, Madeleine Yue Dong, and Tani E. Barlow, 96–119. Durham: Duke University Press.

Thompson, Paul. 1985. "Women in the Fishing: The Roots of Power between the Sexes." *Comparative Studies in Society and History* 27 (1): 3–32.

Uganda AIS. 2012. Uganda AIDS Indicator Survey 2011 Ministry of Health, Kampala, Uganda, and ICF International, Calverton, MD.

UNAIDS. 2005. *AIDS Epidemic Update.* December 2005. Geneva, Switzerland: Joint United Nations Program on HIV/AIDS (UNAIDS) and World Health Organization.

UNAIDS. 2009. *AIDS Epidemic Update.* December 2009. Geneva, Switzerland: Joint United Nations Program on HIV/AIDS (UNAIDS) and World Health Organization.

UNAIDS. 2012. *AIDS Epidemic Update.* December 2012. Geneva, Switzerland: Joint United Nations Program on HIV/AIDS (UNAIDS) and World Health Organization.

UNDP. 2005. *Human Development Report.* New York, NY: United Nations Development Program.

UNDP. 2013. *Human Development Report.* New York, NY: United Nations Development Program.

U.S. Census Bureau 2012. Statistical Abstract of the United States 2012.

Van Damme, Lut, Amy Corneli, Khatija Ahmed, Kawango Agot, Johan Lombaard, Saidi Kapiga, Mookho Malahleha, Fredrick Owino, Rachel Manongi, Jacob Onyango, Lucky Temu, Modie Constance Monedi, Paul Mak'Oketch, Mankalimeng Makanda, Ilse Reblin, Shumani Elsie Makatu, Lisa Saylor, Haddie Kiernan, Stella Kirkendale, Christina Wong, Robert Grant, Angela Kashuba, Kavita Nanda, Justin Mandala, Katrien Fransen, Jennifer Deese, Tania Crucitti, Timothy D. Mastro, and Douglas Taylor for the FEM-PrEP Study Group 2012. "Preexposure Prophylaxis for HIV Infection among African Women." *New England Journal of Medicine* 367 (5): 411–22.

Van der Straten, Ariane, Lut Van Damme, Jessica E. Haberer, and David R. Bangsberg. 2012. "Unraveling the Divergent Results of Pre-Exposure Prophylaxis Trials for HIV Prevention." *AIDS* 26 (7): F13–F19.

Van Maanen, John. 1988. *Tales of the Field: On Writing Ethnography.* Chicago: University of Chicago Press.

Vaughan, Meghan. 1991. *Curing Their Ills: Colonial Power and African illness.* Cambridge: Polity.

Vavrus, Frances. 2003. *Desire and Decline: Schooling amid Crisis in Tanzania.* New York: Peter Lang.

Veblen, Thorstein. 2006. *Conspicuous Consumption. Unproductive Consumption of Goods Is Honourable.* New York: Penguin.

Ware, Norma C., Monique A. Wyatt, Jessica E. Haberer, Jared M. Baeten, Alexander Kintu, Christina Psaros, Steven Safren, Elioda Tumwesigye, Connie L. Celum, and David R. Bangsberg. 2012. "What's Love Got to Do with It? Explaining Adherence to Oral Antiretroviral Pre-Exposure Prophylaxis for HIV-Serodiscordant Couples." *JAIDS: Journal of Acquired Immune Deficiency Syndromes* 59 (5): 463–68.

Watkins, Susan Cotts. 2004. "Navigating the AIDS Epidemic in Rural Malawi." *Population and Development Review* 30 (4): 673–705.

Weinbaum, Alys Eve, Lynn M. Thomas, Priti Ramamurthy, Uta G. Poiger, Madeleine Yue Dong, and Tani E. Barlow, eds. 2008. *The Modern Girl around the World: Consumption, Modernity and Globalization.* Durham: Duke University Press.

Weiss, Brad. 1993. "Buying Her Grave: Money, Movement and AIDS in North-West Tanzania." *Africa: Journal of the International African Institute* 63 (1): 19–35.

Weiss, Helen A., Maria A. Quigley, and Richard J. Hayes. 2000. "Male Circumcision and Risk of HIV Infection in Sub-Saharan Africa: A Systematic Review and Meta-Analysis." *AIDS* 14:2361–70.

Weiss, Robert S. 1994. *Learning from Strangers: The Art and Method of Qualitative Interview Studies.* New York: Free Press.

Whisson, Michael. 1964. *Change and Challenge.* Christian Council of Kenya.

White, Luise. 1990. *The Comforts of Home: Prostitution in Colonial Nairobi.* Chicago: University of Chicago Press.

Whitehead, Clive. 1993. "Education for Subordination? Some Reflections on Kilemi Mwiria's Account of African Education in Colonial Kenya." *History of Education* 22 (1): 85–93.

WHO/UNAIDS/UNICEF. 2011. *Global HIV/AIDS Response: Epidemic Update and Health Sector Progress towards Universal Access 2011 Progress Report.* World Health Organization.

Wiederman, Michael W. 1997. "Extramarital Sex: Prevalence and Correlates in a National Survey." *Journal of Sex Research* 34 (2): 167–74.

Williams, Christine. 1992. "The Glass Escalator: Hidden Advantages for Men in the 'Female' Professions." *Social Problems* 39(3): 253–67.

Wojcicki, Janet Maia. 2002. "Commercial Sex Work or Ukuphanda? Sex-for-Money Exchange in Soweto and Hammanskraal Area, South Africa." *Culture, Medicine and Psychiatry* 26 (3): 339–70.

Wolfe, Tom. 2000. *Hooking Up.* New York: Farrar, Straus and Giraux.

Woodruffe, Helen R. 1997. "Compensatory Consumption: Why Women Go Shopping When They're Fed Up and Other Stories." *Marketing Intelligence and Planning* 15 (7): 325–34.

Yamano, Takashi, and Thomas S. Jayne. 2005. "Working-Age Adult Mortality and Primary School Attendance in Rural Kenya." *Economic Development and Cultural Change* 53 (3): 619–53.

Yeatman, Sara E. 2007. "Ethical and Public Health Considerations in HIV Counseling and Testing: Policy Implications." *Studies in Family Planning* 38 (4): 271–78.

Yngstrom, Ingrid. 2002. "Women, Wives and Land Rights in Africa: Situating Gender beyond the Household in the Debate over Land Policy and Changing Tenure Systems." *Oxford Development Studies* 30 (1): 21–40.

Zabin, Laurie Schwab, and Karungari Kiragu. 1998. "The Health Consequences of Adolescent Sexual and Fertility Behavior in Sub-Saharan Africa." *Studies in Family Planning* 29 (2): 210–32.

*Zambia Demographic and Health Survey, 2001-2002* (ZDHS). 2003. Lusaka, Zambia; Calverton, MD: Central Statistical Office (Zambia); Central Board of Health (Zambia), and ORC Macro.

Zelizer, Viviana. 2000. "The Purchase of Intimacy." *Law and Social Inquiry* 25 (3): 817–48.

———. 2005. *The Purchase of Intimacy*. Princeton, NJ: Princeton University Press.

*Zimbabwe Demographic and Health Survey 2005-2006* (ZDHS). 2007. Harare, Zimbabwe; Calverton, MD: Central Statistical Office (Zimbabwe) and ORC Macro.

*Zimbabwe Demographic and Health Survey 2010-2011* (ZDHS). 2012. Harare, Zimbabwe; Calverton, MD: Central Statistical Office (Zimbabwe) and ORC Macro.

Zukin, Sharon, and Jennifer Smith Maguire. 2004. "Consumers and Consumption." *Annual Review of Sociology* 30:173–97.

# Acknowledgments

In the production of this book, I have benefited from the help of many people both in the United States and in Kenya. In graduate school at the University of Chicago, I thank my dissertation committee, Patrick Heuveline, Linda Waite, Shelley Clark, and Jennifer Cole, for their commitment, guidance, and insight throughout my early years of writing the material for this book. I am especially grateful to Patrick for believing in me and my potential, and supporting me from my beginnings in the program. I am also grateful to Linda for her generosity and kindness to me in my final years of graduate school. For research funding, I thank the Population Reference Bureau, and I also thank Linda Waite and Shelley Clark for supporting my fieldwork in Kenya with their University of Chicago research funds. I am grateful for the Henderson Dissertation Fellowship, which allowed me time to write. I thank William Parish and Edward Laumann from the China research group, along with Omar McRoberts and Andrew Abbott, for many conversations and insights that contributed to my thinking on the subject matters in this book. I am especially grateful for Andy's mentorship in the years after I left Chicago, when this work began its long and winding transformation into a book. During its initial shaping, my work also benefited from critical comments and questions raised by participants of the African Studies Workshop (then run by Jean and John Comaroff, along with Jennifer Cole and Ralph Austen) and Robert Wyrod especially, and the Social Theory and Evidence Workshop, both at the University of Chicago, an American Sociological Association panel in 2007, and critical comments by Francis Dodoo and Parfait Eloudou-Enyegue, the latter of whom, in a workshop that was part of a PRB fellowship, pushed me to consider adding men into my project.

I thank my fellow graduate students in the Sociology Department at Chicago, and in particular, Genevieve Pham-Kanter, Daniel Menchik, and Stefan Bargheer, for their critical comments on my work. Along with them, I thank Erin York Cornwell and Benjamin Cornwell, for their encouragement, friendship, and support, especially in my final year of graduate school. The support and encouragement of my wonderful community of friends and church in Hyde Park sustained me and kept me going; in particular, my weekly coffees over seven years with Jackie Jay, regular hangouts with Jackie Ogutha, Jessy Beauvais, and Shannon Harmon, and weekly prayer meetings with my amazing girls, Shannon Bjorklund and Zuzana Johansen kept my mind, soul, and spirit together. I continue to be grateful for my virtual hangouts with Zuzi and Shan and my almost two-decade-long friendship with Kirsten Spalholz McTernan, who always keeps me laughing.

In the years since leaving Chicago, as the manuscript percolated, my thinking has benefited from both teaching and feedback on different ideas in a number of classes I have taught as an assistant professor at the University of Colorado, Boulder. In particular, I am grateful for the undergraduate students in my classes on Cross Cultural Perspectives on Romantic Relationships, Sociology of HIV/AIDS, and Sex, Gender, and Society, among whom I tried out and refined many ideas in this book, and for the graduate students in Logics of Qualitative Inquiry, among whom I felt pushed to clarify my thinking and writing on issues of method. During the book-writing process, I have benefited from comments on drafts of several chapters in this book. I am grateful for critical comments and feedback from the junior faculty workshop (most of whom are no longer "junior") organized by Christina Sue, whose members were her, Jenn Bair, Jill Harrison, Stefanie Mollborn, Hillary Potter, Isaac Reed, and Amy Wilkins; my Agincourt group, Nicole Angotti, Enid Schatz, and Jill Williams; the

Women and Gender Studies reading group; and James Ogude, Myles Osborne, Janet Jacobs, and Judy Auerbach. A few people read and gave useful feedback on drafts of the manuscript in its entirety. I thank my father, Aloo Mojola, Craig McIntosh, and Patrick Heuveline for their thoughts on the manuscript as a whole. I especially want to thank for their immense intellectual generosity Stef Mollborn (who read it more than once), Sara Yeatman, and Dick Jessor, along with the anonymous press reviewers for their close (sometimes it felt too close!), line-by-line, foot-note-by-footnote comments on the manuscript. Their detailed thoughts and focused attention along with their critiques—especially when I disagreed—immensely improved the quality and rigor of the book, and the clarity of my arguments in it. I thank Judy Auerbach and Christine Williams for their belief in me as a scholar, and the suggestion of Christine Williams that I try California. I am grateful for Naomi Schneider's support of this work, and to her along with Christopher Lura and the rest of the team at the Press (including Chalon Emmons, Robert Demke, and Elena McAnespie), and Betsy Zenz for facilitating the production of this book.

The Department of Sociology at the University of Colorado, Boulder, has been a great environment in which to flourish; it is that rare academic space where exceptional scholarship and intellectual rigor are combined with full and rich lives outside of work. Additionally, the Institute of Behavioral Science has provided a wonderful home for research and writing. I am grateful to have the support of the Health and Society program, as well as the Population program and the NICHD-funded Population Center for space and support to write, colleagues with whom to regularly converse, and opportunities to present my work in progress. Among my many supportive colleagues at CU-Boulder, both senior and junior, I single out a few here. I still remember with gratitude the wonderful welcome to the department I received from the then chair, Mike Radelet, who, along with his family, hosted me, lent me some basic furniture, and, in true Colorado style, lent me a mountain bike, complete with helmet and light, and invited me to join a six-hour group hike in the mountains. My polite (silently culture shocked) decline to the latter then has transformed into an enjoyment of a place where it still feels surreal to live, a place whose beauty and grandeur I grew up seeing in jigsaw puzzles, Christmas cards, and pictures. I feel blessed to have landed here. I thank Jane Menken,

Janet Jacobs, and Dick Jessor for their mentorship, support, encouragement, and belief in me, especially in the early tenure track years when I
was struggling to get papers into print and was unsure about my abilities
as a scholar. I am also grateful to Jason Boardman for his encouragement
to follow my heart and write this book, especially when it felt like a high-
risk strategy. For making my life outside of work full, I have particularly
cherished the friendship of Christi Sue, Fernando Riosmena, and Stef
Mollborn, along with the love, encouragement, and cheerleading support
of my Boulder family: Jayme, Joanne and Eric, Ian, Emily and Kyle, Joam
and Cora, and (the now-not-so-little) Hana.

In Kenya, I am grateful for the permission of the Ministry of Education
of the Government of Kenya, along with the provincial and relevant district and school officials, to conduct this research. I thank my Luo teachers, Bill Ogutu, Lilian, and Jonathan, at the ACK language school in
Nairobi for introducing me in such an enthusiastic manner to the dhoLuo
language. I also thank key informants, Flossie Adoyo, Dr. Joyce Olenja,
Maureen Ong'ombe, Edwin Moyi, Seruya Moyi, Dr. Dan Kaseje, and Alice
Natecho, for their insightful conversations with me as I began my fieldwork. I am also immensely grateful to (the late) Jane Ogwayo, Alice
Otwala, Sam Omollo, Helen Ong'ombe, Jack Ong'ombe, David Manyatta,
James Kambona, Ocholla Ong'ombe, and TICH/Great Lakes University
for going out of their way to help me with the logistics of community
interviews, and for lending me their wisdom and insight. I thank my tire-
less and hardworking research assistants, principally Marian Adongo and,
for the final month, Rose Diang'a, for their company, patience, and help
with this work. I also thank Zedekiah and Joy Otolo and (the late) Tom
and Noel Kibira for their generosity in hosting me, and they, along with
my brother Luka, my uncle Wanga, and my parents, Dr. Aloo and Freda
Mojola, for their many challenging conversations, continued encouragement, love, patience, hope, and faith in me throughout my graduate school
and tenure-track journey. Finally, and most of all, I would like to thank all
my respondents who shared their thoughts and lives with me and hope
that this work will be not only a contribution to knowledge, but also a
contribution to making their lives better and bringing an end to the HIV
epidemic.

# Index

Page numbers in *italics* indicate figures, maps, and tables.

CPSIA information can be obtained
at www.ICGtesting.com
Printed in the USA
JSHW020305231121
20683JS00001B/25